Tenosynovitis
A Case Of Mistaken Identity

Alan Tindall FCII

Iron Trades
Insurance Company Limited

First published in Great Britain in 1993
by
Iron Trades Insurance Company Limited
21-24 Grosvenor Place, London SW1X 7JA

Copyright © 1993 by Iron Trades Insurance Company Limited

ISBN 0-9521676-0-3

Apart from any fair dealing for the purposes of research or private study, or criticism or review, as permitted under the Copyright, Designs and Patents Act, 1988, this publication may not be reproduced, stored or transmitted in any form or by any means, except with the prior permission in writing of the publishers, or in the case of reprographic reproduction in accordance with the terms of licences issued by the Author's Licensing and Collecting Society Limited and the Copyright Licensing Agency Limited. Inquiries concerning reproduction outside those terms should be sent to the publishers at the above address.

The publishers make no representation, express or implied, with regard to the accuracy of the information, advice, opinions or comments contained in this book and cannot accept any legal responsibility for any errors or omissions that may take place.

British Library Cataloguing in Publication Data
CIP data for this book is available from the British Library

Conditions of sale:
This book is sold subject to the condition that it shall not, by way of trade or otherwise, be lent, re-sold, hired out, or otherwise circulated, without the publisher's prior consent, in any form of binding or cover other than that in which it is published and without a similar condition including this condition being imposed on the subsequent purchaser.

Book design by Cats Creative Services Limited

Printed and bound in Great Britain by
Castle Press Limited, St. Leonards-on-Sea, East Sussex

*"Whatsoever thy hand findeth to do,
do it with thy might."*

ECCLESIASTES 9. 10.

TENOSYNOVITIS – A CASE OF MISTAKEN IDENTITY

ACKNOWLEDGEMENTS

Alan Tindall would like to thank
the following people and organisations for their
assistance in the production of this book:

Dr John Blow, Margaret Cahillane, Sharon Davies,
Alexandra Goscombe, Kathryn McCarthy, Pat Smith and Bryan Jepp of
Iron Trades Insurance Company Limited

Alistair Cook and Peter Smith of
Meridian Marketing Resources Limited

Yvonne Dixon BA (Hons) PGCE

Chris Goldhawk

Contents

	PAGE
PREAMBLE	9
INTRODUCTION	14
DEFINITIONS	
– CONDITIONS	19
– MEDICAL TERMS	24
INCIDENCE	30
MECHANISM OF THE UPPER LIMBS:	
– STRUCTURE & FUNCTION	38
PATHOLOGY	46
PSYCHOSOCIAL FACTORS	48
TYPE OF COMPLAINT:	
– CLINICAL FEATURES	51
– CLINICAL DIAGNOSIS	52
– DESCRIPTION OF COMPLAINT	53
CAUSE OF UPPER LIMB DISORDERS:	
– OCCUPATIONAL RISK	69
– BIOMECHANICAL FACTORS	70
– UNSAFE SYSTEMS OF WORK	71

TENOSYNOVITIS – A CASE OF MISTAKEN IDENTITY

	PAGE
CONTROL & MANAGEMENT:	
– TREATMENT	73
– PREVENTION & RISK REDUCTION	74
PRESCRIPTION & OFFICIAL GUIDANCE:	
– PRESCRIPTION	86
– OFFICIAL GUIDANCE	92
UPPER LIMB DISORDERS: SUMMARY & CONCLUSIONS	98
STATUTORY DUTY	100
INVESTIGATION & CLAIMS HANDLING	109
LITIGATION & CASE LAW:	
– THE CONDUCT OF THE REASONABLE & PRUDENT EMPLOYER	120
– A REVIEW OF CASE LAW	121
– THE IDENTIFIABLE LEGAL ISSUES	139
– DAMAGES: EXAMPLE OF COURT AWARDS	139
ADVICE & GUIDANCE TO EMPLOYERS	148
RESEARCH PUBLICATIONS/REFERENCES	154
APPENDIX	160
INDEX	162

FOREWORD

It is strange but nonetheless true that a number of medical conditions now covered by the all embracing title of "Upper Limb Disorders" are conditions that have been known about for decades but are still causing much misunderstanding and confusion in relation to their diagnosis and cause. On the employment scene there is little guidance available to assist employers in combating work related injuries of this type despite there being a fairly major problem in a variety of industries.

It was primarily for this reason that we felt there was a need to commission a thorough review of the subject and produce a consolidated, definitive document to assist in dealing with some of the major issues.

As a company with many years of experience in employer's liability insurance we would have been concerned if we were unable to produce such a document ourselves. Alan Tindall, a senior official at our North East office based in Leeds, was therefore commissioned to undertake the work. We hope it will be found that the result is a very comprehensive study of the subject that will be of assistance to all those who are concerned with the problem and in particular will offer much guidance to employers in preventing this type of medical condition. The Iron Trades Insurance Company Limited is a great believer in prevention, for cures are not always possible once damage is done.

Apart from employers and in particular our own policyholders, we hope that the work will also be of assistance to others in the insurance, medical and legal professions.

Many thanks to Alan Tindall for his efforts. Dr John Blow, our medical adviser, a member of the Faculty of Occupational Medicine, gave much appreciated advice on the medical issues.

Bryan Jepp
General Manager (Commercial Insurances)

Tenosynovitis – A Case Of Mistaken Identity

PREAMBLE

As awareness of occupational hazards increases, today's employers must devote an increasing amount of time to dealing with the precise requirements imposed by legislation in the expanding area of health and safety.

Considering the plethora and depth of legislation in the last 30 years, most people might be forgiven for thinking that workplace reform is a relatively recent concept, the result of a diligent Factory Inspectorate pursuing the wishes of concerned public opinion, of improved technical and medical research and of having a Government committed to improving working conditions throughout industry.

It is not often realised that the origins of reform are sometimes much more distant.

Consider the latest complaint which has emerged to cause problems for the insurance market.

The onset of aches and pains in the arms following heavy and prolonged labour has been known for a long time – under many different names but to most people as tenosynovitis even if the term is technically inaccurate.

Over a century ago when the early pioneers of industrial reform were beginning to make some impact upon the grim realities of factory life, the authorities of the day produced a report that contained the following passage:-

> "That excessive fatigue, privation of sleep, pain in various parts of the body, and swelling of the feet experienced by young workers, coupled with the constant standing, the peculiar attitude of the body, and the peculiar motions of the limbs required in the labour of the factory, together with the elevated temperature and the impure atmosphere in which that labour is often carried on, do sometimes ultimately terminate in the production of serious, permanent, and incurable diseases, appears to us to be established".

TENOSYNOVITIS – A CASE OF MISTAKEN IDENTITY

Although the measures that were subsequently adopted and made law (by the Factories Act of 1833) were aimed largely at restricting the employment of young persons in industry, that extract from the Report of the Factories Inquiry of 1833, placing emphasis on "excessive fatigue" and "the peculiar motions of the limbs required in the labour of the factory" reveals a surprising degree of foresight in the light of modern research.

Arguably therefore factory owners, if they had troubled to read the report, were already aware of the possibility of serious and permanent damage to the upper limbs from the factory process although it is doubtful whether this aspect of the report received any significant publicity.

One who had troubled to investigate the factory process more closely was the Leeds medical pioneer Dr Charles Turner Thackrah who published in 1831 his essay on the Effects of the Principal Arts, Trades and Professions on Health & Longevity. This work made frequent reference to **bad occupational postures** as a source of disability. Particularly interesting are the comments on the textile trade:-

> "We see no plump and rosy tailors: none of fine form and strong muscle. The spine is generally curved. Pulmonary consumption is also frequent. Let a hole be made in a board of the circumference of the tailor's body, and let his seat be placed below it. The eyes and the hands will then be sufficiently near his work: his spine will not be unnaturally bent, and his chest and abdomen will be free".

An early view of ergonomics perhaps!

Even the 18th century was not without its medical pioneers. Bernardino Ramazzini, often described as the father of occupational medicine, wrote in his published work The Diseases of Scribes and Notaries:-

> "Incessant driving of the pen over paper causes intense fatigue of the hand and the whole arm because of the continuous and almost chronic strain on the muscles and tendons, which in the course of time results in failure of power in the right hand".

Complaints arising from the excessive use of the hand and arm were certainly known therefore before the onset of the industrial revolution.

Preamble

Reviewing the history of occupational health a century or so later one of the diligent factory inspectors John C Bridge commented that the most striking feature seemed to be the long period that elapsed before the science of medicine was considered necessary as an aid to improving working conditions in industry.

Much has changed.

Occupational health is now at the forefront of industrial reform. Much medical and scientific research has been written and published. Ergonomics is no longer thought to be some form of strange incurable disease. Advice to employers is plentiful.

We must therefore examine the likely sources of advice for employers. They may for instance belong to trade organisations who frequently are prepared to offer advice and guidance to their members. The Health & Safety Executive with its many specialist sections is another helpful source of information. There are increasing numbers of industrial consultants of various kinds who are happy to meet a growing demand for technical advice – at a price. There are many specialist publications on the market. Even the trades unions now publish their own health and safety advice.

In the midst of this avalanche of information, what of the role of the insurer?

Employer's liability insurance has been compulsory since 1972. It cannot legally be avoided. Premiums have to be paid; claims must be met. Insurers therefore have a considerable interest in attempting to reduce the risks likely to give rise to claims.

Insurers can offer other services. The insurance industry through the activities of specialist companies and brokers has for many years operated safety and/or risk assessment services providing (often free) assistance and guidance through the wealth of modern legislation, especially where alternative advice would have been too difficult or too costly to follow.

Guidance on systems and practices may necessitate an appraisal of the employer's legal position. With our experience of handling claims in conjunction with specialist firms of solicitors, we are well placed to offer practical guidance to help reduce the employer's liability based on legal precedent.

In reviewing the very many forms of upper limb disorder, including that of tenosynovitis, we examine the historical background, the problems of definition and the current stance of the medical and legal professions. Attention is drawn

TENOSYNOVITIS – A CASE OF MISTAKEN IDENTITY

to the pitfalls involved in defending legal liability claims in a rapidly growing area of litigation.

The section on case law is in part taken from our own experience in handling common law claims – we accept that there may be other cases which have been contested or settled but which have not been reported or received any publicity and some which have attracted media attention which were settled out of court. It is important to have in mind that a court is only able to pronounce on the evidence before it. If the proper evidence is not adduced the outcome is unpredictable and probably unfavourable to the employer. Employer's liability insurance is very much a specialised subject.

Employers operating in shops and offices should not assume that the risks relate only to factory premises. Indeed, insurance companies are as much affected by the new Regulations on display screen use as the employers to whom they often preach.

Employers should assess their own position carefully. The benefits of a fully fit workforce, fewer claims and reduced premiums are obvious.

This book is designed to assist employers and others towards an in-depth understanding of the subject and we recommend that it is read in full. Each section is also designed to stand on its own as far as possible and in such circumstances some repetition is unavoidable. However, any reader wishing to concentrate on the practicalities of the subject only, may wish to turn to the chapter entitled "Control and Management of Upper Limb Disorders" as a starting point.

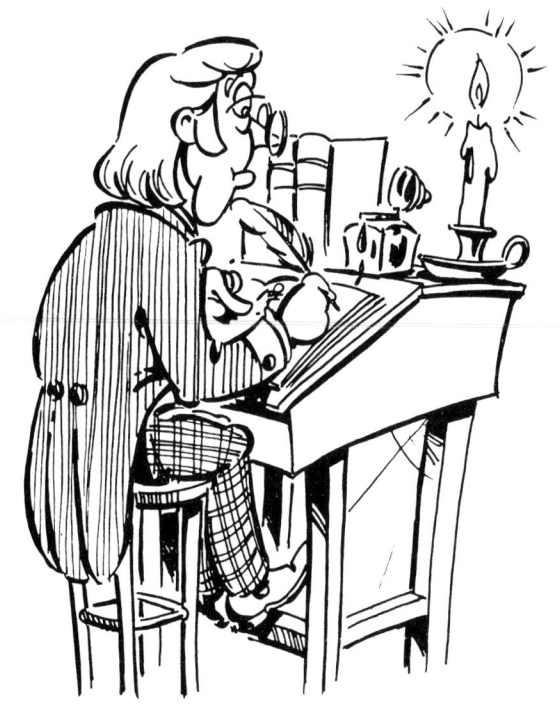

ADVANCEMENT YES, BUT THE REAL PROBLEMS ARE NO DIFFERENT.

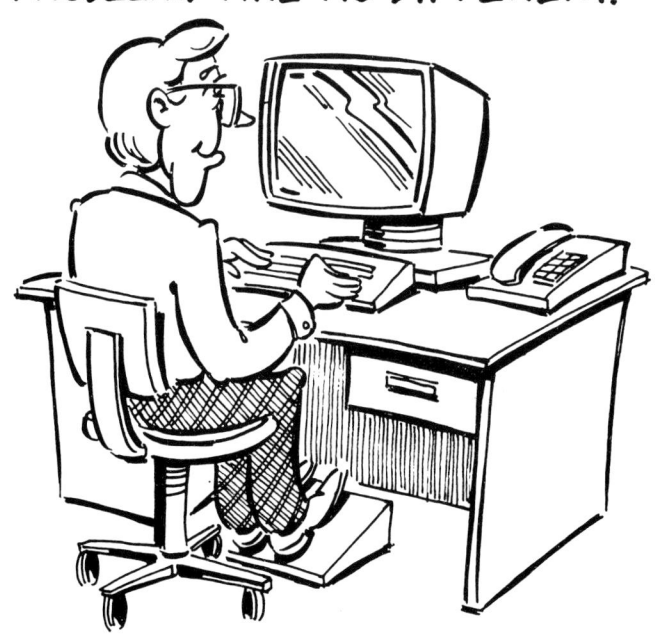

INTRODUCTION

Upper limb disorders allegedly caused by repetitive tasks are occupational health problems of increasing significance to employers and insurers.

The combination of repetitive upper limb exertion, static posture and mental as well as visual stress characterises much of modern work. This characteristic has resulted from an increasing mechanisation and specialisation in many common industrial and commercial tasks. Innumerable repetitive tasks can be found in factories and offices – from production line techniques to keyboard operation.

Employer's liability insurers have for many years handled claims from employees suffering from a form of wrist complaint known as tenosynovitis – or **teno** as it is commonly called.

Many people are aware of someone who has suffered or is suffering from **teno** and in the last decade or so compensation claims have become common without any real thought having been applied to the definition.

How then should **teno** be defined and when should the term be used?

Defined accurately, tenosynovitis is but one of a wider and increasing group of hand and arm soft tissue conditions which during the 1980's became popularly known as repetitive strain injuries and which are now perhaps more accurately beginning to be called upper limb disorders.

Tenosynovitis used as a general term covering the wider range of hand and arm complaints is imprecise both medically and descriptively and where used inaccurately is capable of causing confusion in the precise area of litigation. So to a lesser extent is the more popular "repetitive strain injury". Recent guidance from the Health & Safety Executive prefers the term "upper limb disorder".

Conditions arising from upper limb disorder, whether caused by repetition or otherwise, can be painful and are sometimes disabling but in most cases the effects are trivial – provided that early action is taken to deal with the complaint in the form of rest and/or treatment. Upper limb disorders **often** occur quite independently, without any occupational origin.

Introduction

Whilst most occupational injuries result from a clearly defined event or accident, upper limb disorder may gradually develop over a period. In some instances the early symptoms of disorder may not occur whilst the employee is working – the link with work activity may not even be realised.

Some upper limb disorders arise from activity associated with ordinary movement – what may make such activity hazardous is prolonged repetition often in a forceful and awkward manner without rest or recovery time. Where it can be proved that there is a relationship with work activity there is, if early action to deal with the problem is not taken, potentially a high cost – to employers in terms of time lost, to insurers from resulting claims.

There are additional related costs which include:-

- sick pay
- higher insurance premiums resulting from compensation
- decreased production/productivity through sickness
- increased workload and stress on remaining employees
- cost of short-term contract working
- loss of training investment
- discomfort to the individual
- secondary effects on the individual's family.

It is therefore unwise to overlook early signs of complaint however trivial they may seem in the belief that the problem will disappear. There have been a number of well publicised recent cases where employees whose complaints were ostensibly ignored have obtained substantial compensation through the courts having convinced the authorities that their disorder was occupationally related and little or no relief was obtained by complaining to the employer.

A good example was the much publicised settlement of £45,000 for a "typing related disease" in 1989.

Regardless of such publicity there is however no easy route to compensation. There is no discounted compromise "scheme" to which a complainant might have recourse such as those applicable in claims arising from noise induced hearing loss or vibration white finger set up by Iron Trades Employers Insurance Association Limited and followed by other insurers. In claims arising from upper limb disorder, each claim must be treated on its merits – causation and liability must be proved.

Tenosynovitis – A Case Of Mistaken Identity

Not all claims will succeed, nor will compensation where it is justified necessarily be high. Awards such as the example given are exceptional and relate to specific circumstances. They by no means represent the general level of compensation available. There are many more cases of mild injury without long spells of absence from work. In any event damages cannot replace the importance of avoiding injury.

Nevertheless with growing awareness and publicity some members of the public may be tempted to endeavour to relate their occupation to all the many common musculo-skeletal aches and pains that exist as part of the activities of daily living. There is little doubt that back, neck and arm pain is common. At any given time nearly a tenth of the adult population has pain in the neck or arm or both and one in three have had it at some time. In the average person there is no necessity to look for any specific reason. It only remains to have the condition medically defined.

It is not always appreciated that in pursuing compensation, problems can arise for the potential claimant at the outset. Most claimants refer to their condition as tenosynovitis or tennis elbow but insurers should insist upon a correct diagnosis of the alleged complaint.

The problem of incorrect definition and diagnosis is not necessarily confined to insurers. For instance tenosynovitis is alleged to be the second commonest prescribed disease in the United Kingdom (HSE Guidance Note MS 10) but the accuracy of the statement needs close examination given true tenosynovitis is supposedly a condition diagnosed only **rarely** by medical practitioners.

The source of that inaccuracy (and by implication the starting point for many of the legal cases now arising) is most probably the certificate issued by general practitioners who, whatever the vague nature of complaints presented, and whatever diagnostic signs are present, will frequently write on the certificate **tenosynovitis** not because they are unaware or do not have an understanding of the more ill-defined upper limb disorders but because that is the name by which wrist complaints have come to be known.

The potential claimant then presents himself to the local DSS office and becomes a **statistic**. In a recent High Court judgment, Jupp J emphasised the problem by the following words – "It is probable that many varied and uncertain diagnoses relating to the hand and forearm have been lumped together to give rise to this alarming and provocative statistic".

Alternatively such action may be quite deliberate because **tenosynovitis** is

INTRODUCTION

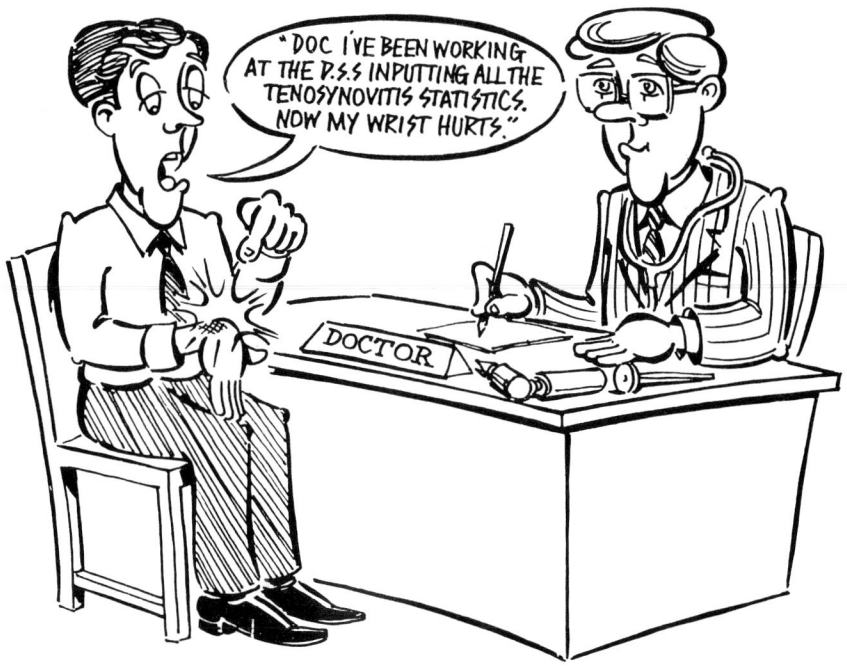

one of the few conditions which can be compensated under DSS Regulations.

Where the problem is not confined to the wrist, the diagnosis is usually **tennis elbow** for the same reasons (although tennis elbow is not compensatable under present DSS Regulations) thus ignoring all the many other elbow and upper arm conditions that exist.

Consequently the average worker is often conditioned to the view that the complaint is occupationally caused even before additional pressure to pursue a claim against the employer is exerted by working colleagues, trades unions or the local newspaper advertising the services of specialist solicitors for this type of claim.

Despite recent research and much publicity the aetiology of the condition remains mysterious and the difficulties of defining such disorders, diagnosing them correctly and providing appropriate treatment have resulted in a considerable amount of confusion. There remains no common agreement on a name for the problem. Instead there are many collective names which refer to a range of conditions. Such labels cover a variety of afflictions which have some common ground – pain, disablement, repetition – but are often misleading. One possible explanation for the **apparent** recent increase in this

Tenosynovitis – A Case Of Mistaken Identity

type of case may be an increase in **reporting** rather than **in incidence**. Many unions report a significant increase in upper limb disorder cases in recent years although this probably reflects greater expectations on the part of union members and more awareness about the adverse effects of work on health.

That the number of new reported cases (and by implication claims) is growing, there is little doubt – whether this be due to increased awareness, intensified publicity or simply jumping on the bandwagon. There are other factors:-

- increasing exposure to new technology
- mechanisation and specialisation
- change of environment or work process
- change in philosophy
- increased militancy in the traditionally passive area of the white collar workforce.

The true reason for the apparent increase probably lies in a combination of factors. The issues however are worthy of careful consideration.

DEFINITIONS – CONDITIONS

There are numerous collective terms in use for the range of conditions characterised by persistent discomfort or pain in muscles, tendons and other soft tissues with or without physical manifestations.

Why there should be so much variation in the terminology used is not easy to understand. Those who apply the descriptions – usually medical specialists or other research experts – normally take great care in the choice of words when defining a particular condition or problem precisely for the purpose of avoiding ambiguity.

A review of the medical and other contemporary literature however shows a wide degree of variation in the expressions that are used to define a multitude of hand and arm conditions many of which have the same basic meaning. Whilst to some extent this may reflect the thinking and approach in different countries (given that this is a problem not exclusively confined to the UK) it may equally be taken to highlight the disagreement on the likely cause.

What is apparent is that it is a **misconception** that such conditions are **usually** caused or aggravated by work and associated **mainly** with repetitive motion as it is perfectly clear from the literature that risk factors are non-occupational as well as occupational.

Many of the terms in current use **imply** damage and task related causality even before corroborating evidence is available. Defendants would be wise to guard against an enthusiasm for this trend and to use terms that are less emotive and medically more accurate rather than some of the pseudo-scientific labels describing what may be nothing more than musculo-skeletal pain of undetermined diagnosis.

Repetition by itself ignores other important factors such as **force** (undesirable forceful movement), **static loading** (sustained or constrained awkward posture), frequency, duration and speed. Static loading is the work

Tenosynovitis – A Case Of Mistaken Identity

that the muscles must do to hold the body or parts of it in certain positions for a sustained length of time. It may require more energy than movement and is demonstrated by holding the arms outstretched or above the head. Any modest length of time in that position will produce discomfort.

Many tasks require the above three elements – therefore discomfort is common.

It is also widely believed that susceptibility, predisposition and psychosocial or psychological factors including stress in the working environment may contribute although among the experts there remains considerable disagreement. Consequently definition remains a contentious issue and in purporting to define the precise nature of the disorders, each of the collective terms in current use may to some extent be misleading.

Terms in Current Use

Several relatively wide definitions are used to describe the range of hand and arm conditions which may have a work related element. Frequently a similar descriptive phrase is used with only a slight change of wording or emphasis. Where this applies the change is acknowledged. The list is not necessarily exhaustive.

Repetitive Strain Injury (RSI)

Also known as repetition strain injury, repetitive strain syndrome or disorder and occupational repetitive motion injury.

This term was first used in Australia in the early 1980's to describe a number of ill-defined symptoms of arm, neck, shoulder, hand or wrist pain predominantly reported by office workers. The term has subsequently found support in this country.

The classification of RSI with the commonly acknowledged over-use conditions of the upper limb is however misleading and serves as an example of the confusion that may be caused by the random use of doubtful terms.

For instance the terms emphasise repetition at the expense of force and posture. Use of the term RSI **assumes** repetition is the cause and **assumes** the result is physical injury but there is no scientific evidence that repetitive

DEFINITIONS

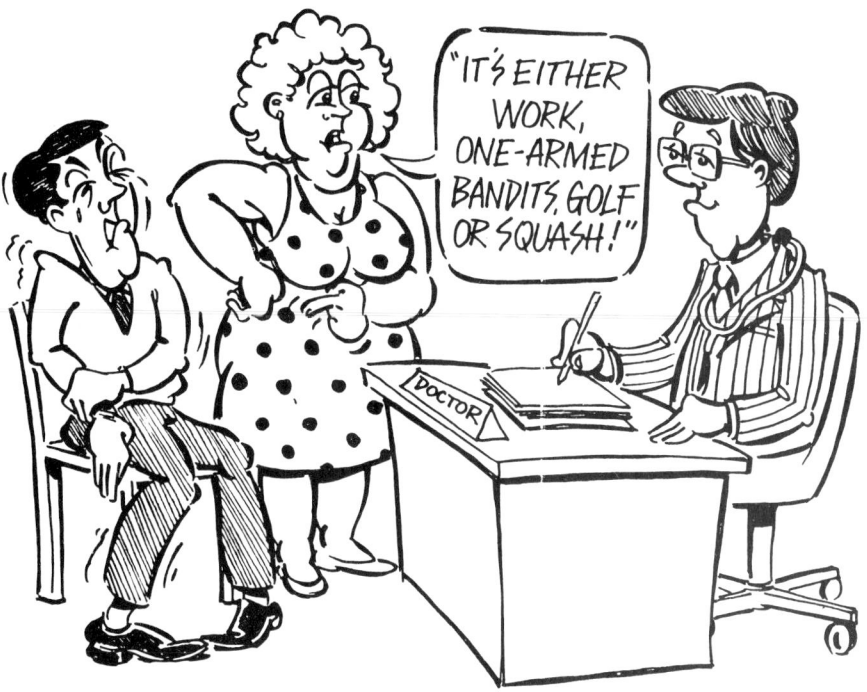

movement always causes tissue strain nor that strain automatically leads to injury.

Strain implies damage to tissue but often there is no objective physical abnormality in the upper limb other than tenderness. Ancillary investigation is frequently negative; no signs of tissue damage such as swelling, bruising, redness and increased temperature can be found.

Pain is often alleged but on investigation may not follow any known neurological pattern.

RSI is a form of fatigue but unlike ordinary muscle fatigue. The term muscle fatigue, in an unscientific lay sense, is commonly used to describe the results of unaccustomed muscular activity more usually described as muscle ache or tiredness. Normally this can be expected to subside within 48 hours of stopping such activity. It is certainly not known to persist many years after discontinuing the activity. This is often the reported experience of alleged RSI sufferers.

It is important therefore to distinguish RSI from the common perception of fatigue and over-use conditions. There is evidence that RSI is a multi-factorial, socio-economic problem with a major psychological basis, not a true physical condition resulting from injury; it may become a firmly established neurosis by the time a specialist opinion is sought. Subsequent treatment may then require the patient's acceptance of a psychological contribution to the condition. It will be clear from this that avoidance of the term RSI is preferable.

Musculo-Skeletal Disease (Musculo-Skeletal Disorder)

A general term covering a multitude of muscle and bone disorders in which hand and arm complaints are prominent.

Over-Use Injury

Frequently described as muscle over-use syndrome or over-use tendon injury. The implications of the description are obvious. Occupational over-use syndrome is a biased term – it is implicit in this description that occupation is the major factor in the complaint.

Tenosynovitis

Frequently used (incorrectly) as a general term to describe a whole range of disorders of the arm and wrist and is the term preferred by General Practitioners and other doctors. Tenosynovitis is however a specific complaint involving inflammation of the synovial sheath of the tendon and is only **one form** of upper limb disorder.

Upper Limb Strain Injury (ULSI)

A frequently used term. More accurate in its description of upper limb disorders than RSI but has the same implications.

DEFINITIONS

Upper Limb Disorders (ULD)

The terms adopted by the Health & Safety Executive in its recently published Guidance are **Work Related Upper Limb Disorders (WRULD)** or simply **Upper Limb Disorders (ULD):** deliberately vague expressions used to describe a range of different conditions affecting the soft tissues of the hand, wrist, arm and shoulder. Less frequently, similar conditions may affect the lower limbs.

Sometimes the expression **upper limb soft tissue disorders** may be used.

NB *The Guidance Note specifically states that although in recent years the term **repetitive strain injury** has been commonly used, it is medically imprecise and not sufficiently accurate to cover the conditions observed.*

It may therefore be advisable to follow the Guidance using **upper limb disorder** (or even simply **disorder**) as a descriptive term. Where it appears in an occupational context it is intended to mean Work Related Upper Limb Disorder associated with repetition, force and posture.

Other Terms In Use

The following terms have also been used in published literature:-

- muscle related upper limb pain
- pain of undetermined diagnosis
- repetitive trauma
- upper extremity disorder (discomfort).

In the USA the preferred term is **Cumulative Trauma Disorder** or alternatively Cumulative Trauma Injury.

Japan and Sweden prefer the expression **Occupational Cervicobrachial Disorder**.

The latest suggestion to emerge from Australia is **Reversible Fatigue Syndrome**.

These expressions cover a multitude of different complaints – there are many variations.

DEFINITIONS – MEDICAL TERMS

Medical terminology can be confusing. Some of the common medical terms in use and which may be met when considering medical evidence are described.

Abduction   Movement away from the body's mid-line. In the case of the thumb, movement away from the plane of the palm.

Adduction   Movement towards the mid-line. In the case of the thumb and fingers, movement towards the long finger (middle of the hand).

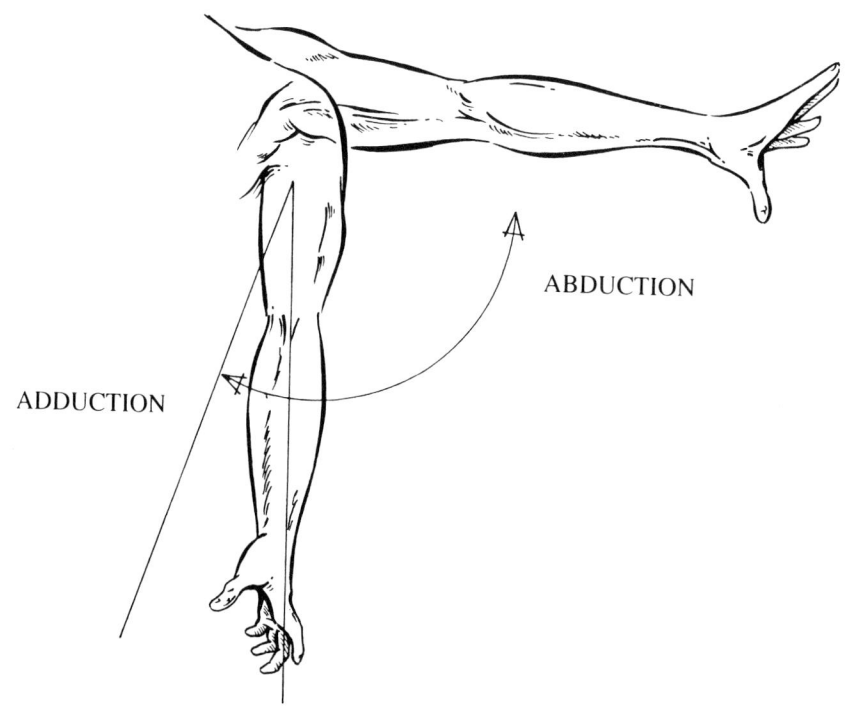

Definitions

Carpal Tunnel A channel in the wrist through which pass a number of tendons and the median nerve.

Cartilage A hard pliant substance covering the end of every long bone where it forms a joint with other bones (articular cartilage). It is sometimes found in combination with fibrous tissue, as in vertebral discs.

Cervical Pertaining to the neck.

Chuck Grip The three point grip formed by opposing the thumb, index and long finger tips.

Crepitus A slight creaking or grating sound heard or sensation felt resulting from the rubbing together of two rough surfaces such as in osteo-arthritis of a joint or the broken ends of a bone. It may also occur in "dry joints", within muscles, or where a roughened tendon moves through an inflamed tendon sheath.

Diagnosis Determination of the nature of a disease by investigation of its signs, symptoms and history.

Dorsiflexion Movement of a joint in a backward direction.

Dysfunction Mechanical malfunction of the musculo-skeletal system involving the production of pain or discomfort normally accompanied by loss of joint range and muscle power.

Epi A prefix meaning situated upon or outside of.

Epicondylitis Inflammation of the epicondyle of the elbow occurring where the muscles join the bone at the elbow causing pain, swelling and discomfort.

Extension The term applied to the process of straightening or stretching a limb (opposite to flexion).

Tenosynovitis – A Case Of Mistaken Identity

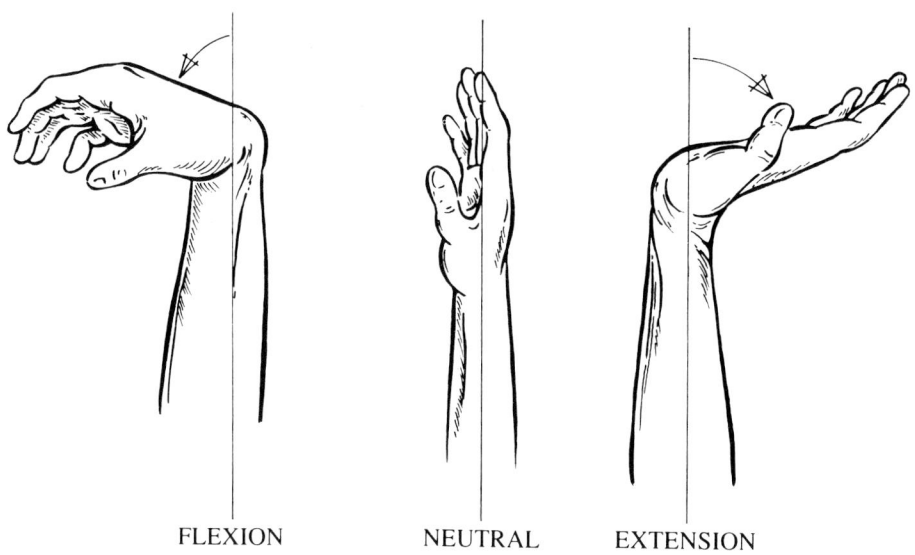

FLEXION　　　NEUTRAL　　　EXTENSION

Finkelsteins Test	A test for diagnosis of de Quervain's tenosynovitis whereby the hand with the thumb held within the clenched fingers is passively forced into ulnar deviation producing pain over the radial styloid.
Flexion	Moving a joint into the bent position (opposite to extension).
Ligaments	Strong bands of fibrous tissue which bind together the bones that enter a joint. They are in some cases cord-like, in others flattened bands – most joints are surrounded by a fibrous capsule in which capsular ligaments are incorporated. Ligaments restrict movement but are elastic within narrow limits.
Palmar Flexion	Moving the wrist in the direction that the palm faces.
Paraesthesia	An abnormal sensation such as a tingling feeling – the familiar "pins and needles".

DEFINITIONS

Peri A prefix meaning around.

Periarthritis Inflammation around the joint due to infection or injury, causing pain and restricted movement.

Peritendinitis (or Crepitans) Traumatic inflammation of the tendons of the hand and forearm or of the associated tendon sheath when the site of the lesion is in the tendons above the upper limit of the tendon sheath.

Phalens Test A test for provocation of numbness and paraesthesia by median nerve compression over the carpal tunnel during active wrist flexion and held for one minute.

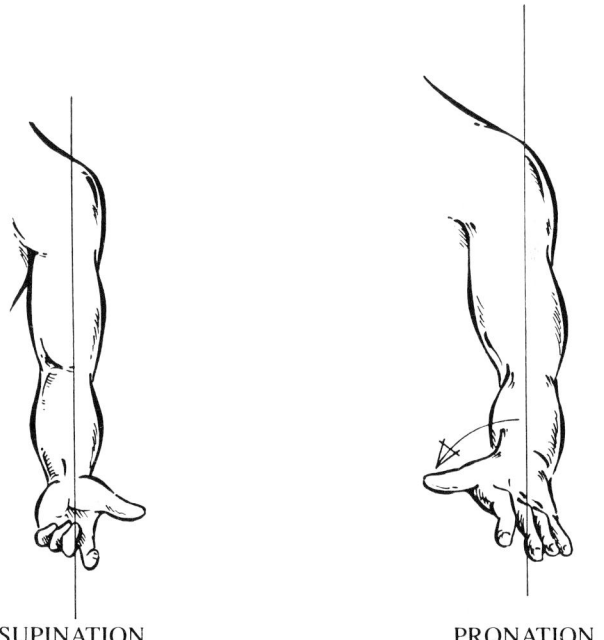

SUPINATION   PRONATION

Pronation Twisting the forearm to bring the palm of the hand facing downwards (opposite to supination).

Sprain The tearing or stretching of ligament fibres attached to a bone when a joint is moved beyond its normal range.

Tenosynovitis – A Case Of Mistaken Identity

Stenosis The term applied to a condition of abnormal narrowing in any passage or orifice of the body.

Strain The stretching and possible tearing of some of the fibres in a muscle as a result of excessive movement or activity.

Supination Twisting the forearm to bring the palm of the hand facing upwards (opposite to pronation).

Synovial Membrane The lining of the cavity of a joint.

Synovitis Inflammation of the membrane lining the joint cavity. Usually painful and accompanied by effusion of fluid within the synovial sac.

Tendon The cord that attaches the end of a muscle to the bone or other structure upon which the muscle acts when it contracts. Also known as the sinew or leader.

Tendovaginitis (or tenovaginitis) Inflammation of a tendon and of the sheath which surrounds it (sometimes used as an alternative to tenosynovitis).

Teno A prefix meaning related to a tendon.

Tenosynovitis (or Tenositis) Inflammation of a tendon sheath and possibly the tendon.

Definitions

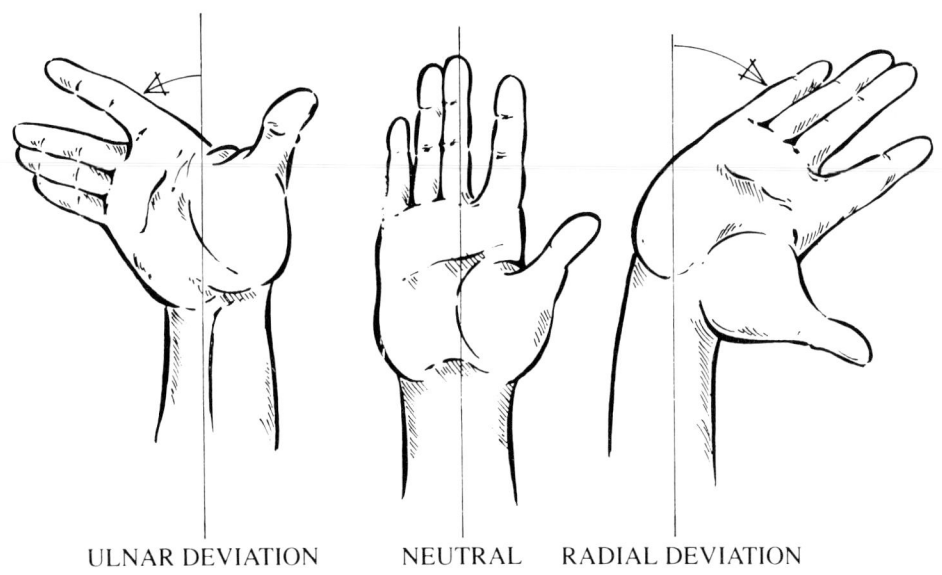

ULNAR DEVIATION　　NEUTRAL　　RADIAL DEVIATION

INCIDENCE

The statistical measurement of occupational ill health presents two basic problems:-

1. Defining what is meant by occupational ill health.
2. Determining the number of cases falling within the definition.

The existence of occupational disability has always been recognised in common speech by such terms as housemaids' knee, boilermakers' deafness, farmers' lung, firemen's or glass workers' cataract and hoppers' gout – all specific conditions relating to vulnerable occupations.

Less well known, perhaps are expressions such as weavers' bottom, hatters' shakes, Billingsgate hump, nuns' bursitis and potters' rot but the implications of such descriptions are obvious.

Many such terms refer specifically to conditions of the hand and arm – these include milkers' arm, scriveners' palsy, telegraphists' cramp, writers' cramp, lumberjacks' finger, tailors' callosities – indicative of the fact that the origins of hand and arm complaints lie in the traditional occupations of the past and these complaints are not necessarily a result of the application of modern techniques.

Workers today suffering from occupational upper limb disorder fall into two broad categories:-

- industrial workers
- office workers.

Historically the complaints were involved with repetitive manual work in certain crafts and over the years there have been reports of an increased incidence in such traditional areas as:-

- tobacco and tea packers (Conn 1931)

INCIDENCE

- agricultural workers (Pozner 1942)
- filing and assembly work in the car industry (Thompson & Plewes 1951)
- braiders in ropemaking (Smiley 1951)
- hop picking (Hunter 1955)
- carpenters, upholsterers and linoleum fitters hammering nails (Hunter 1955)
- core making and ramming (Wilson 1956).

The 1965 report of H M Inspector of Factories refers to the following occupations as having specific risk of upper limb disorder:-

- packeting of food
- typing
- comptometer operating
- sewing machining
- chicken preparing
- metal and wood-working
- gardening
- hop picking
- upholstering
- net and grommet making.

The 1970 report of H M Inspector of Factories adds the following:-

bricks	- hand making, handling, laying
chickens	- eviscerating, trussing, packing
engineering	- press operating, light assembly
	- food preparation for canning
	- boot and shoe industry
	- furniture manufacture.

However, it was not until November 1972 that the Department of Employment published the first official guidance on tenosynovitis and related conditions under the heading **C E M A Guidance Note 5 – Beat Conditions/Tenosynovitis.** The Note suggests that tenosynovitis is an important cause of sickness absence. It occurs in many industries but especially

Tenosynovitis – A Case Of Mistaken Identity

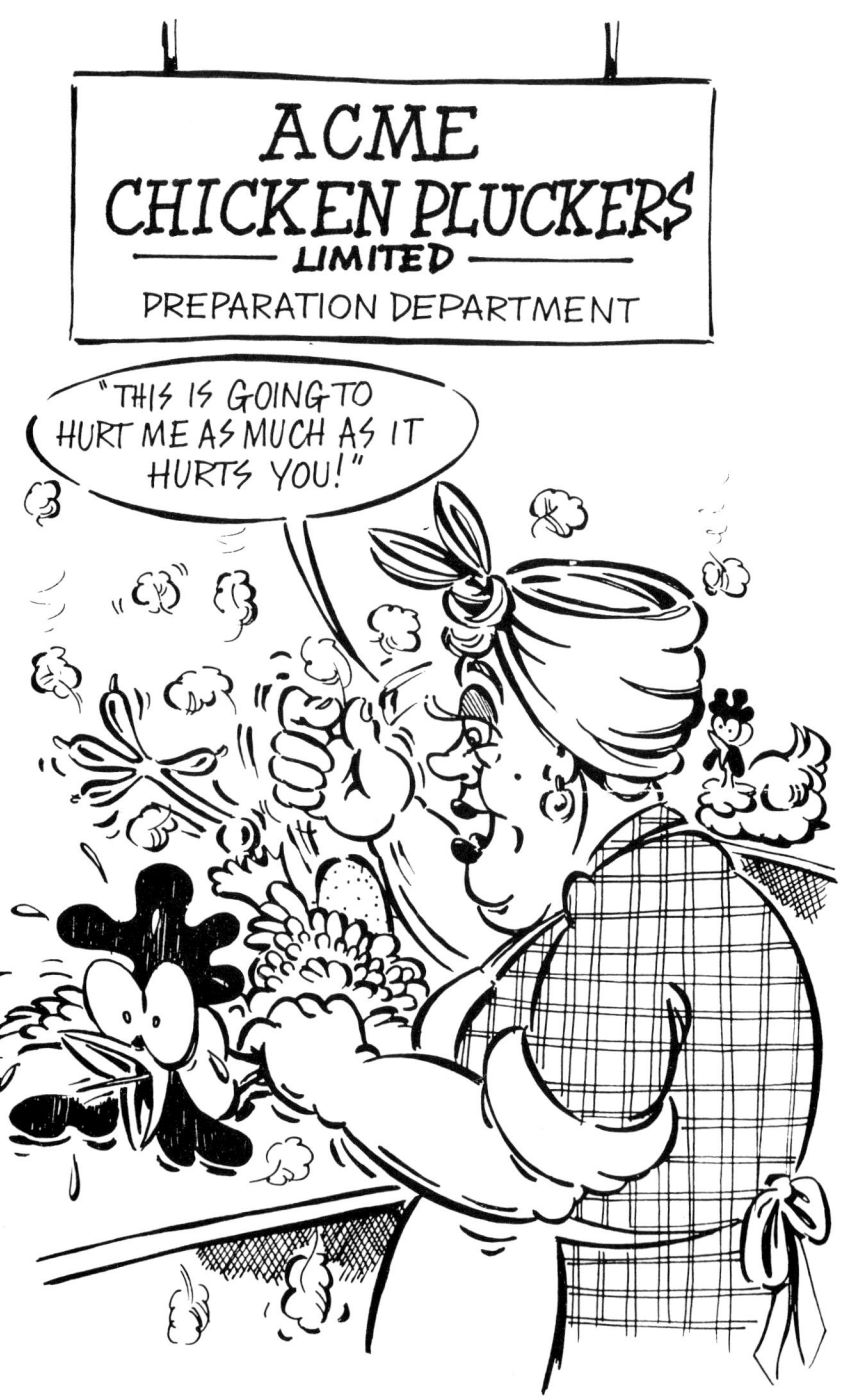

INCIDENCE

those where rapid, repetitive twisting and gripping movements are common such as pottery, glaze dipping, brick making, assembly line work, belt conveyor sorting for food canning, press operations and the evisceration and trussing of chickens.

Guidance Note MS.10 issued in September 1977 follows the earlier report almost word for word suggesting that tenosynovitis is the second commonest prescribed disease in the United Kingdom.

A report by Elenor in 1981 identified six industrial categories having a particularly high prevalence of **repetition strain injuries**:-

1. Electronics industry eg telecommunications assembly.
2. Manufacture of domestic appliances involving mechanical assembly.
3. Poultry processing and packing.
4. Clothing, carpet and bag manufacture requiring manual sewing.
5. Manufacture and packaging of small consumer products eg biscuits, cigarettes and sports goods.
6. Cleaning operations involving heavy scrubbing and polishing machines.

A more recent report (Institute of Occupational Medicine, Edinburgh 1988) suggests that people who work as keyboard operators, cleaners, hairdressers or machine operators are at greater risk of sustaining damage to the soft tissue in their arms, hands and wrists than those in other occupations.

The true prevalence of the disease is unknown.

A report in 1990 by the **University of Birmingham** commissioned on behalf of the Health & Safety Executive suggests that injuries referred to as Repetition Strain Injuries have increased markedly probably because of (not despite) **mechanisation** due to emphasis on:-

- higher rates of repetition
- segmentation and specialisation
- work pacing
- incentive schemes
- concentration on particular points of the anatomy.

The increasing application of computer technology suggests that even larger

Tenosynovitis – A Case Of Mistaken Identity

numbers of keyboard operators may be at risk in the future. It is also reasonable to assume that all those in occupations which include the above features may be at risk.

Under the current reporting system there is no reliable way of finding out what proportion of the workforce suffers from upper limb disorder or the types of work where it may be most prevalent.

Upper limb disorders are not diseases reportable to the Health & Safety Executive under current regulations and the only reliable data are the statistics presented by the Department of Social Security for cases of occupational disease awarded benefit under the Industrial Injuries Scheme. Under these regulations an award may only be made for a **prescribed** disease, that is one which is included in Schedule 1 of the Social Security (Industrial Injuries)(Prescribed Diseases) Regulations 1985.

Apart from beat conditions there are only two **prescribed** upper limb disorders:-

PD.A4   Cramp of the hand or forearm due to repetitive movements.

PD.A8   Traumatic inflammation of the tendons of the hand or forearm or of the associated tendon sheaths.

The following table shows the number of benefit awards made in the 10 year period from 1977 to 1987.

	\multicolumn{5}{c}{Injury & Disablement Benefit}	\multicolumn{5}{c}{Disablement Benefit}
	1977/1978	1978/1979	1979/1980	1980/1981	1981/1982 (10m)	1982/1983	1983/1984	1984/1985	1985/1986	1986/1987
Tenosynovitis and related conditions	3537	3259	3009	2413	2282	1433	337	390	619	289

The majority of these claims were for PD.A8 (commonly referred to as **tenosynovitis**) thus giving rise to the allegation that **tenosynovitis** is the second most common industrial disease (behind dermatitis).

The reliability of these statistics is distorted by benefits rule changes in April 1983 and October 1986 which resulted in a fall of more than 50% in the number of claims made. In April 1983 injury benefit for claimants was replaced by

INCIDENCE

Statutory Sick Pay. From October 1986 disablement benefit is paid only for cases of disability assessed at 14% or more although disabilities from more than one condition can be aggregated to qualify.

There are additional factors which affect the reliability of the statistics:-

1. The ratio of claimants to affected non-claimants is unknown as is the ratio of this type of injury to **other upper limb disorders** which are not included in the statistics even though some may be occupational in origin.

2. There is no scope for inclusion of neck or shoulder disorders which may affect the arms and hands.

3. The self employed are not included under the Industrial Injuries Scheme so the number of awards will understate the actual incidence of occupational disease.

4. There may be substantial under-reporting based either on acceptance or expectation of soft tissue disorders or on a refusal to believe that anything was wrong despite the evidence.

In contrast there is no clear evidence of over-reporting.

These statistics do not provide an adequate guide to national incidence of occupational upper limb disorder, nor do they relate disorders to occupational factors which may have caused them.

Recent comments by the Health & Safety Executive on the health and safety statistics for 1988/1989 express concern over the problems caused by musculo-skeletal disease. They suggest that the last available figure for disablement benefit (1985/86) can clearly be depended upon to offer evidence of the scale of the occupational element of the disease.

However the true incidence of occupational upper limb disorder is almost certainly under-reported.

In 1990 the Labour Force Survey conducted by the Office of Population, Census & Surveys included a special health and safety supplement commissioned by the Health & Safety Executive. The Health & Safety Commission Annual Report for 1990/91 states, "It is possible to have a considerable degree of confidence that the Labour Force Survey generally provides an accurate basis for estimating real levels of work-related injuries." The Labour Force Survey data is of particular interest in providing an indication

Tenosynovitis – A Case Of Mistaken Identity

of the individual's perception of work-related health.

Analysis of relatively small samples requires some caution but based on this survey a startling picture emerges. Specifically discounting upper limb disorders it has been estimated, according to the returns made, that over half a million cases of general musculo-skeletal disorders were attributed to work related causes and a further quarter million cases were allegedly made worse by work. Analysis of upper limb disorder alone revealed 50,000 cases attributed to work related causes with an additional 10,000 cases made worse by work.

Based on such figures, the real incidence of work related disease is clearly much higher than the number of benefit claimants would suggest.

According to the 1988 Institute of Occupational Medicine report, about 9% of upper limb disorders reported to orthopaedic clinics nationally involved the occupations of keyboard operator, cleaner, hairdresser and machine operator.

The 1990 report by the University of Birmingham suggested that the DSS List of Prescribed Industrial Diseases should be reviewed to include those disorders which were identified as work related.

This suggestion was accepted by the Industrial Injuries Advisory Council who recently published their findings. In the event they recommended only the inclusion of carpal tunnel syndrome – they were unable to recommend prescription of any other work related upper limb disorder. Significantly however prescription of carpal tunnel syndrome is recommended on an individual "case by case" basis, that is where the condition can be proved clinically rather than epidemiologically to be related to workplace exposure.

This approach represents a departure from the current parameters of the prescription process.

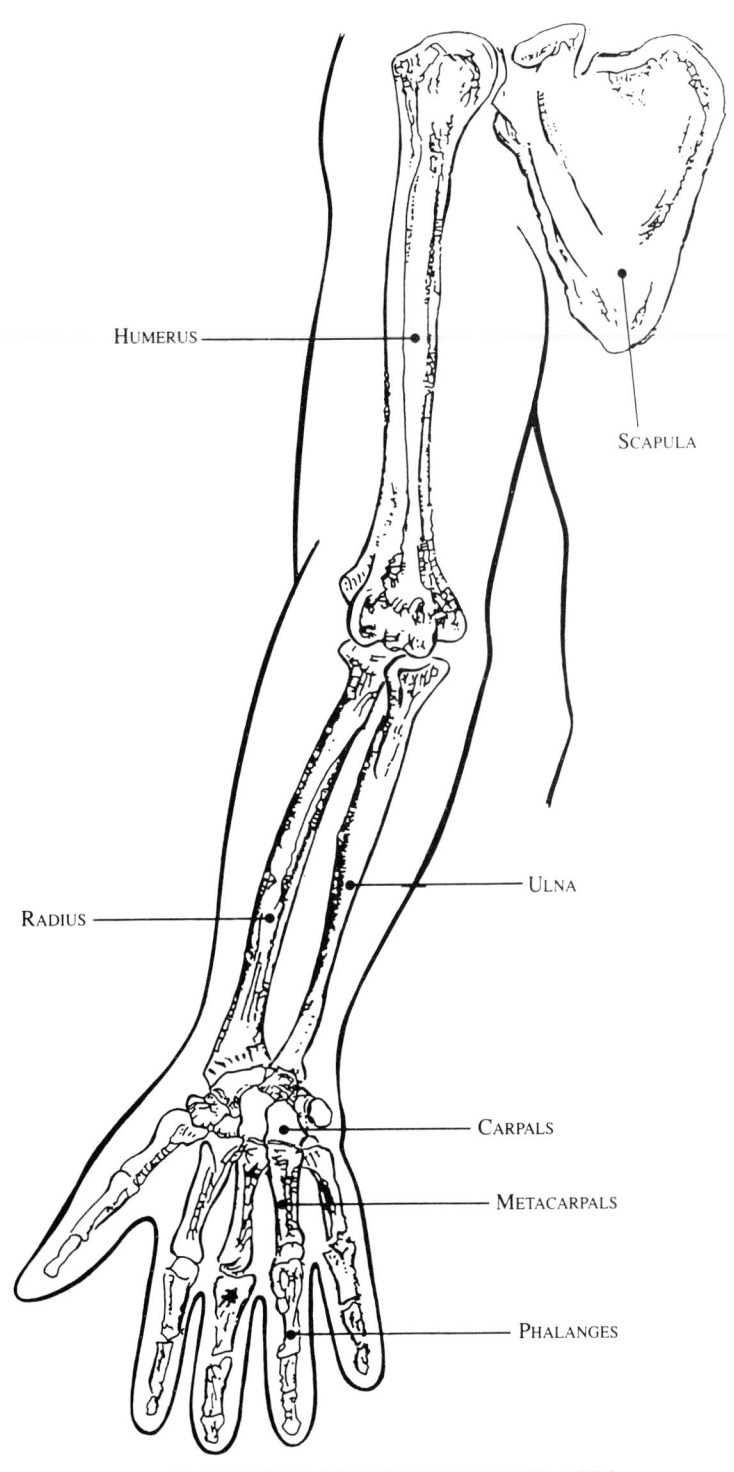

MECHANISM OF THE HAND AND ARM

Mechanism Of The Upper Limbs

Structure And Function

Knowledge of the means by which the human body accomplishes movement is helpful to understanding the more complex nature of its disorders.

A joint or articulation occurs where two or more bones, usually covered with articular cartilage, meet, allowing a variable degree of movement.

Joints are divided into three classes:-

1. Fibrous.

2. Cartilaginous.

3. Synovial.

In a fibrous joint the surfaces of the bones are fastened together by intervening fibrous tissue and no appreciable movement is possible. An example is the bones of the adult skull.

In a cartilaginous joint the opposing bone surfaces are covered with cartilage and joined together by a complex fibrocartilage. Strong ligaments connect the bones but do not form a complete capsule round the joint. The joint between vertebral bodies is an example of a cartilaginous joint.

Synovial joints include most joints in the body; all joints in the arm and leg are synovial. In these:-

- adjacent bone surfaces are covered with cartilage but not attached to each other
- the joint is surrounded by a capsule
- the capsule is lined by a synovial membrane which secretes a lubricating fluid

Mechanism Of The upper Limbs

- the bones are connected by ligaments which may be thickenings in the capsule or superficial to it
- varying degrees of movement are possible depending on the anatomy of the joint and ligaments.

Various other structures, for example muscles and tendons, help to strengthen a joint and limit excessive movement.

The upper limb is an amazingly versatile unit capable of a wide range of movement, is exceptionally strong for its size, is able to undertake delicate and precise manipulation and yet is strong enough to damage itself.

Motion and leverage for the upper limb is provided by muscles and tendons at three major joints – shoulder, elbow and wrist. Movement tends to be limited by ligaments.

Shoulder

The shoulder is the joint formed by the upper end of the humerus and the scapula (shoulder blade). Surrounded by a loose fibrous capsule and strengthened by bands of ligaments the shoulder's main strength comes from the powerful muscles that unite the upper arm with scapula, clavicle and ribs. The shoulder is an example of a ball and socket joint which allows a free range of movement in all directions.

THE SHOULDER
- Clavicle
- Scapula
- Humerus

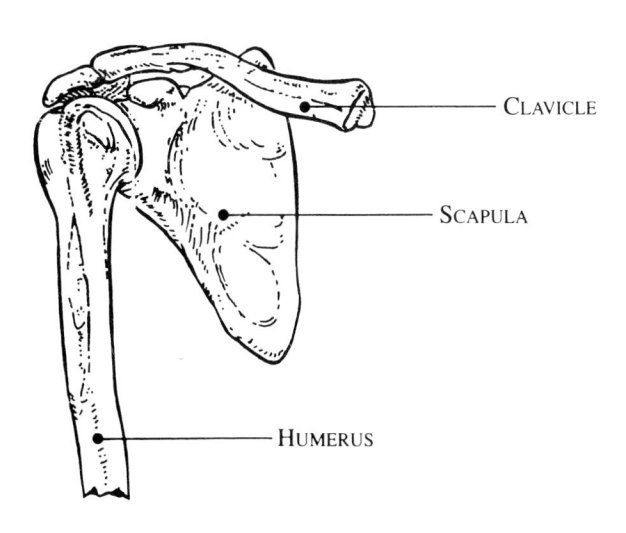

Tenosynovitis – A Case Of Mistaken Identity

Elbow

The elbow is a complex joint in which the forearm bones of the radius and ulna articulate with the humerus of the upper arm.

The joint is capable of two important movements, a flail-like backward and forward movement of the radius and ulna moving in unison against the humerus and a rotary movement of the radius on the ulna and humerus as the palm is turned to face up (supination) or down (pronation).

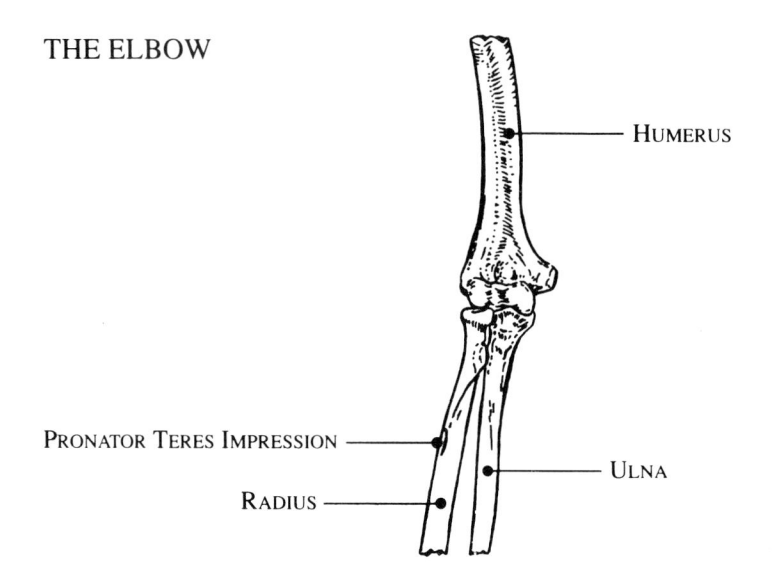

THE ELBOW

- HUMERUS
- PRONATOR TERES IMPRESSION
- ULNA
- RADIUS

The joint is secured at the sides by strong lateral ligaments and at the back and front strengthened by the tendons of strong muscles. The ulnar nerve passing down the forearm has an exposed position behind the inner edge of the humerus at its lower end and is popularly known as the "funny bone".

Wrist

The wrist is the joint in which the lower ends of the radius and ulna articulate with the carpus which consists of eight small bones connecting the bones of the forearm with the metacarpals and phalanges (fingers).

Mechanism Of The Upper Limbs

The movements of the wrist are mainly those of a hinge but it is capable of some movement in every direction.

The carpal bones are closely bound to one another by short, strong ligaments. Three of the carpal bones – the scaphoid, lunate and cuneiform – form the lower surface of the wrist joint, whereas the radius and a triangular shaped cartilage covering the end of the ulna form the upper surface. The two surfaces are united by strong outer and inner lateral ligaments whilst powerful tendons passing through the wrist to the hand and fingers give the joint a large measure of strength.

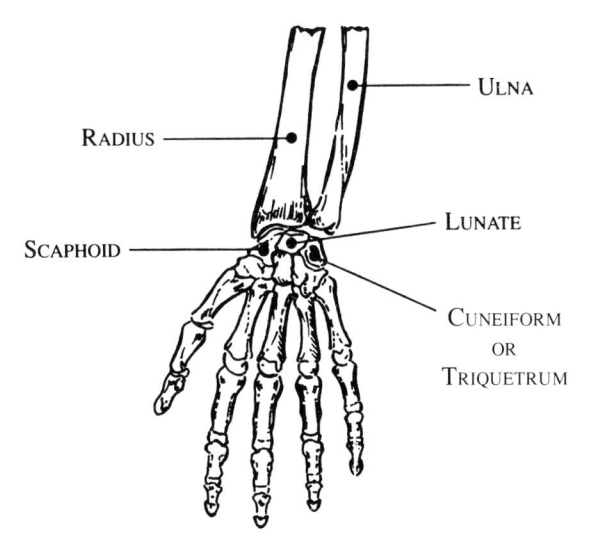

THE WRIST

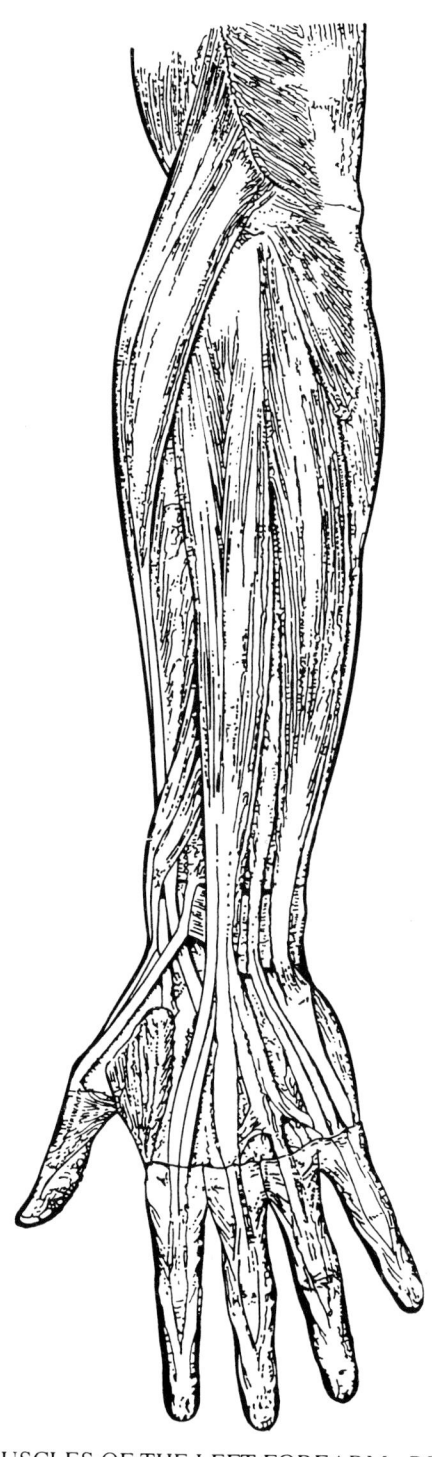

SUPERFICIAL MUSCLES OF THE LEFT FOREARM : POSTERIOR SURFACE

Mechanism Of The upper Limbs

General Function Of The Hand

The hand of man is more highly developed in its structure and in its nerve connections than the corresponding structure in any other animal. The possession of a thumb which can be opposed to the other fingers for **grasp and pinch** is one of the distinguishing features of the human race.

The nerve supply to the hand is connected with a large area on the surface of the brain and is capable of a high degree of fine movement and manipulation; in cases where the brain degenerates, the use of the hand deteriorates particularly early.

Strength, movement and sensation are the three basic requirements that enable the hand to function effectively.

The application of **strength** is brought about by the capacity of muscles to move joints.

Any deficiency of **movement** in any joint of the hand will mean some impairment of manual capacity: either strength, dexterity or both.

There are two types of movement:-

- The **coarse** movements of the fingers, such as those used in gripping large objects, rely for their strength on muscles situated in the forearm ending in strong tendons passing in front of the wrist and through the palm to the fingers and thumb. There are nine tendons at the front of the wrist kept in place by a strong band of ligament known as the flexor retinaculum and partly enclosed in complicated synovial sheaths.
- The **fine** movements of the fingers and thumb – those concerned with dexterity and agility – whilst dependent on the muscles of the forearm are largely controlled by the **intrinsic** muscles of the hand. The action of these small muscles produces the intricate movement of the fingers and thumb.

Sensation, particularly tactile sensation (that relating to the sense of touch) is more important in the hand than in any other part of the anatomy. The hand cannot be used effectively for any operation unless it possesses the capacity for feeling and recognising the object handled. The hand is thus richly supplied with nerve filaments corresponding with its highly specialised function.

Tenosynovitis – A Case Of Mistaken Identity

Sensation to the thumb, index, middle and adjacent half of the ring finger with that part of the palm that corresponds to these digits is supplied by the median nerve. The inner one and a half fingers and the corresponding part of the palm receive their nerve supply from the ulnar nerve. The radial nerve supplies part of the back of the hand on the thumb side.

Damage to any nerve will result in varying degrees of weakness of the affected muscles, even total paralysis both of forearm and intrinsic muscles if the nerve is completely divided at or above the elbow. Nerve damage situated low in the forearm may cause little impairment of coarse gripping capacity as the forearm muscles which carry out this function receive their nerve supply above the level of the injury and hence they can work with normal strength. There will however be loss of dexterity and agility through inability of the intrinsic muscles to carry out their particular functions.

The thumb is by far the most important of the digits – indeed it is generally accepted that at least one half of the manual capacity of the hand is attributable to the thumb. Total loss of the thumb is equivalent in manual capacity to the loss of all the fingers.

In normal use the combination of all these structures together with the complex system of channels contained within the structure allow the tendons within the hand and wrist – controlling the movements of the hand when the muscles are relaxed or contracted – a high degree of freedom and movement that would be difficult to reproduce in any equivalent machine.

As almost all work requires the constant and active use of the arms and hands – frequently unprotected – the structures of the upper limb are very vulnerable to soft tissue injury.

Mechanism Of The upper Limbs

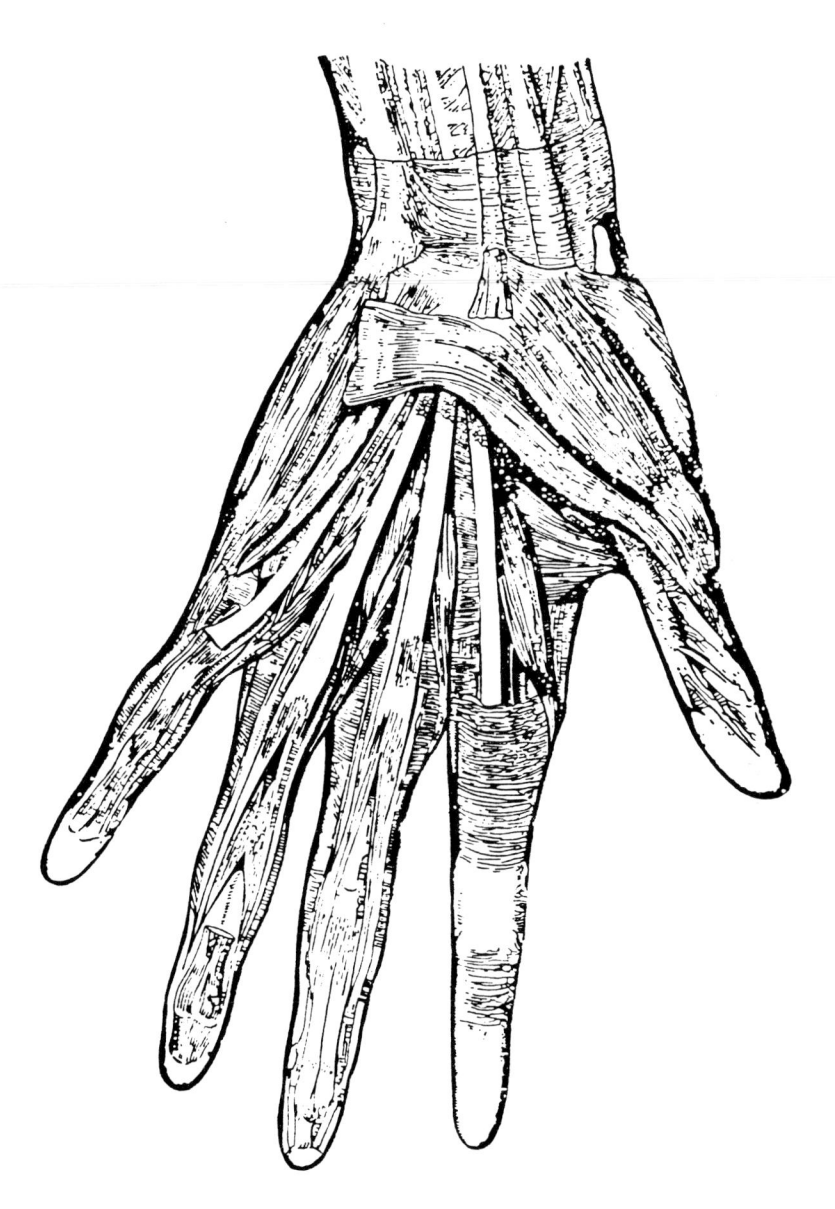

MUSCLES OF THE LEFT HAND : PALMAR SURFACE

PATHOLOGY

Pathology is the science which deals with the structural and functional change caused by disease.

The scientific basis of modern medicine requires that disease should relate to a pathological process which, if it cannot be identified, at least has a rational hypothesis or explanation, enabling appropriate management measures to be undertaken.

Some conditions of the hand and arm have no clearly understood pathology. The relationship between movement and force and the manner in which posture contributes to the development of upper limb disorder remains unclear. The probability is that injury develops from initial inflammatory change with oedema resulting from mechanical and physiological response of the tendons and sheaths to stress.

Repeated sprains and strains (terms often used to describe over-exertion injuries) may produce a pattern of tissue inflammation that is often the forerunner of chronic injury. A permanent disability is sometimes the final result.

Inflammation is a natural response of the body to injury or physical stress. The healing processes of the body can often repair the damage completely if the inflammation is halted early.

The musculo-skeletal system is well able to produce repeated motions at low force levels. Undesirably high force levels may however be imposed on muscles, tendons and joints by some job demands and working practices. Such stresses are usually within the physical capacity or strength of the tissues provided the forces are of short duration and rest periods are adequate. Prolonged tissue loading caused by static posture or performance of very frequent exertions can however be harmful resulting in a diminished functional capacity. Where static posture is combined with awkward movements, musculo-skeletal discomfort will be compounded.

A further factor to be considered is the length of time that the movement or

PATHOLOGY

repetition continues.

Work is a combination of degrees of all these factors.

There is some common ground that upper limb disorders have their origin in **fatigue**. This was described more than two centuries ago, when it was suggested that "incessantly driving pen over paper" caused intense fatigue of the whole arm due to continuous strain on the muscles and tendons eventually resulting in failure of power to the hand.

The relationship of fatigue to discomfort and that of discomfort to injury is however less clear, and there is yet no real agreement on the point at which **damage** occurs to muscles, joints or other tissues.

Work, whatever its nature, is to a degree tiring. Constrained static sitting or standing postures combined with mental and/or visual stress are often inherent in prolonged or repetitive tasks which can rapidly lead to fatigue. Whilst thorough assessment of the risk may enable steps to be taken to remove the sources of extreme and avoidable fatigue, it would nevertheless be surprising if fatigue or at the very least discomfort were not experienced on some occasion.

In order to hold even a fixed position the muscles need to maintain contraction over a period of time resulting in a reduced level of blood to the muscle tissue – this can cause tiredness, cramp and pain.

Fatigue may serve as a warning. Muscles have a sophisticated metabolism and are much more likely to react before other tissues such as tendons. Those prepared to heed such warnings should as a matter of course reduce the pace of their work or alternatively report complaining muscles to the appropriate authority when it is likely that they will be advised to slow down, rest, change their occupation or seek medical advice before the onset of any more serious disorder.

The question of remedy and advice will be more fully discussed later.

PSYCHOSOCIAL FACTORS

Psychology is that branch of medical science which deals with the mind and mental operations especially as they are shown in behaviour.

Ergonomic deficiencies alone are usually not sufficient to generate reports of upper limb disorder – frequently the amount of freedom, control and job satisfaction may be as important as postural factors and increasingly so as the worker gains in experience. Generally the more repetitive the task the more monotonous it becomes, and monotony makes for difficulty in concentration although attention must be concentrated on the task to avoid mistakes.

The contradiction between monotony and concentration demands considerable mental effort and in the absence of any degree of control over the job by the operator it is easy to understand how such tasks can quickly lead in a susceptible person to anxiety, stress, depression and anger.

There is a body of belief – particularly medical – that a psychosocial or psychological element is present in many claims that are presented for upper limb disorder.

Ireland in his 1988 paper "Psychological and Physical Aspects of Occupational Arm Pain" emphasised the psychological aspects of the disorder. He concluded that strain injury bears the "hallmarks of a sociopolitical phenomenon, rather than a medical condition, which on historical precedent will decline when this basis of repetitive strain injury is generally accepted".

Colin Mackay (Health & Safety Executive) thinks most problems could simply be those of fatigue or stress. It is psychological or mood factors that encourage complaints regarding what would otherwise be normal and accepted fatigue after a day's work and which can even be responsible for causing an actual physical lesion. In this regard he accepts that psychological stress can cause muscle stress and tension which in turn will aggravate symptoms of muscle fatigue to such an extent that injury may be either caused or at least claimed.

Bell, writing in the Medical Journal of Australia, calls repetitive strain injury

Psychosocial Factors

an **iatrogenic epidemic of simulated injury** ie he suggests that it can be created by the way doctors diagnose and treat aches and pains which result from unaccustomed exercise. He concludes that "the experience (in Australia) has the appearance of a major medical blunder".

In Australia, claims to have lowered the incidence of repetitive strain injury have not been verified and coincide with an increased medical awareness of the psychological aspects.

In this country, a leading consultant orthopaedic surgeon suggests there are symptoms of arm pain of many kinds for which there are no medical signs and for which no cure has been found by the profession. The cause may initially be unknown but because the perceived risk is in the work, psychological pain develops without any basis in reality.

According to Ireland it is not surprising therefore that redress in the form of compensation benefits proves more palliative than many rehabilitation programmes.

The argument that psychological or psychosocial factors have **any** bearing on the cause of upper limb disorder is not **universally** accepted by all specialists. Many ergonomists do not accept this. Neither do the trades unions and their legal advisers. The contrary argument is that the evidence that physical disability caused by upper limb disorder is associated with psychosocial factors is limited.

It appears unlikely that non-physiological hypotheses could explain all musculo-skeletal problems reported – such hypotheses do not diminish the need to correct any ergonomic deficiencies present.

Tenosynovitis – A Case Of Mistaken Identity

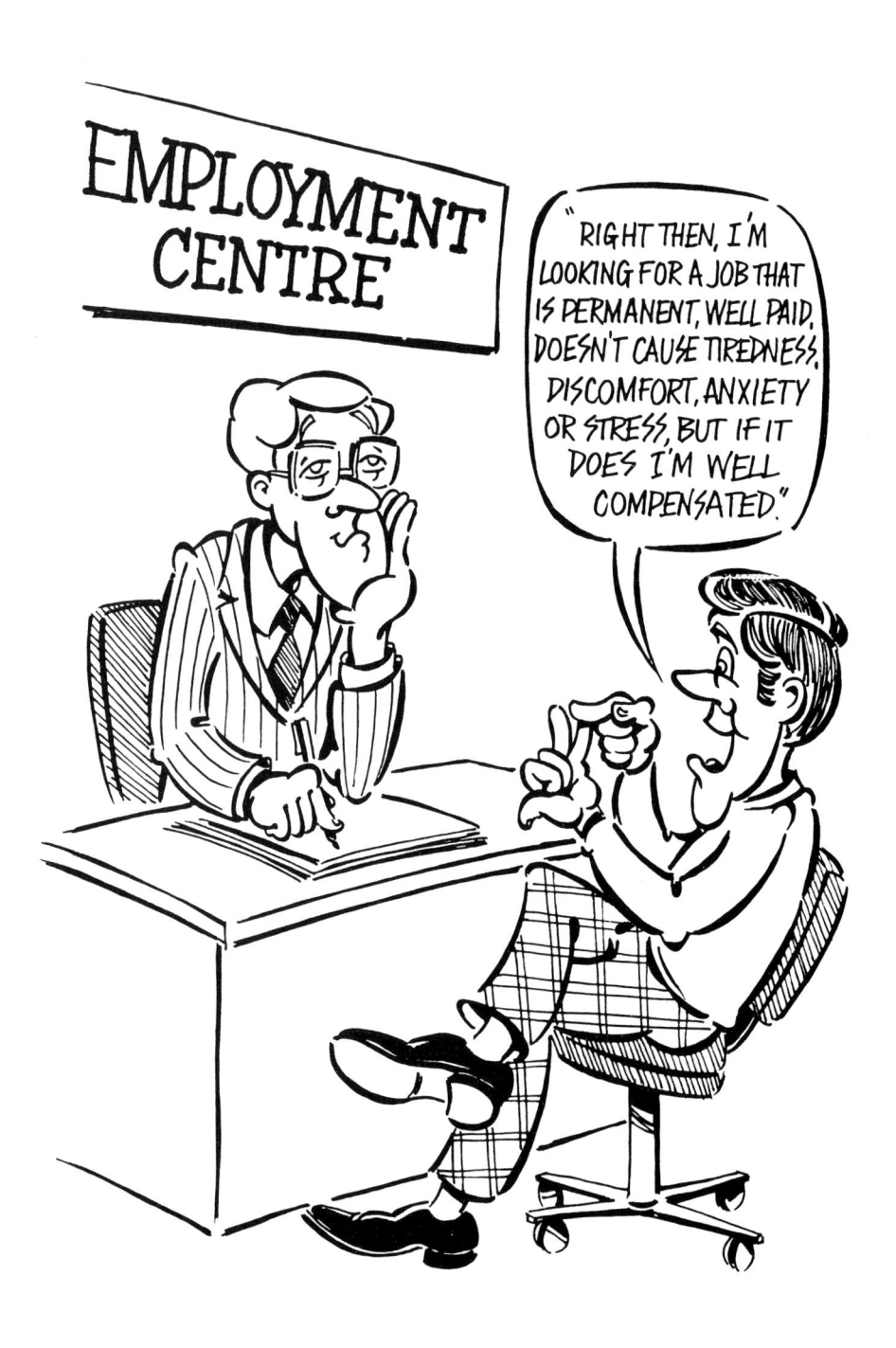

TYPE OF COMPLAINT

The human hand is a valuable industrial resource – some would say the most valuable. Most people take for granted the strength and versatility of the upper limbs – and abuse them accordingly.

Aching limbs will however sooner or later react and all too often the end result is pain, functional disability and immobilisation of the affected parts.

This may be as much due to age, as lifestyle and occupation; studies have invariably shown that frequency and severity of symptoms quite often involving both hands increase with age not, with recreational or occupational hand activity.

Nor is disability necessarily confined to the female population as is so often thought to be the case. It just so happens that more females are employed in occupations likely to give rise to these kind of symptoms. This includes employment in the home.

There are however many examples among the male population – not necessarily due to housework.

This section looks briefly at the features that may result from upper limb abuse – whether from age, lifestyle, occupation or recreation – in either gender, the steps in diagnosis and the main complaints arising highlighting the importance of taking all reasonable steps to protect the health and safety of this most valuable resource.

Clinical Features of Upper Limb Disorder

In general, clinical features are varied and widespread but may include some or all of the following:-

- aching or painful fingers, arms or wrist and pain in the elbow on certain movements
- discomfort

Tenosynovitis – A Case Of Mistaken Identity

- tenderness
- soreness/stiffness
- weakness (difficulty in gripping objects)
- swelling
- numbness or tingling in the fingers, hands or wrist
- paraesthesia
- functional disability (restriction or loss of movement).

The latent period is normally short. Onset may be gradual or sudden. Symptoms can be persistent.

Clinical Diagnosis

Should have regard to the following:-

- clinical and occupational history
- physical examination
- consideration of non-occupational causes.

There are three main categories of diagnosis:-

- patients in whom the diagnosis of an upper limb disorder is beyond doubt, for example in peritendinitis crepitans
- patients who have genuine problems that they believe mistakenly to be caused by their job
- the bandwagon effect, namely those patients who are well aware that symptoms are not due to occupation but who hope to establish such a relationship.

Accurate diagnosis is often impossible.

Type Of Complaint

Description of Complaint

Manifestation of upper limb disorder takes many forms, and in general terms conditions can be grouped under the following headings:-

- hand and wrist
- forearm and elbow
- shoulder and neck.

The following medical descriptions apply to the most important of these conditions:-

Hand and Wrist

- carpal tunnel syndrome
- de Quervain's disease
- Dupuytren's contracture
- gamekeepers' thumb
- ganglion
- occupational cramp
- tenosynovitis
- trigger finger/thumb (stenosing tenosynovitis crepitans).

Forearm and Elbow

- epicondylitis (tennis/golfers elbow)
- peritendinitis crepitans
- pronator teres syndrome
- radial tunnel syndrome.

Shoulder and Neck

- bicipital tenosynovitis
- bursitis (of the shoulder)
- capsulitis
- rotor (rotator) cuff syndrome or supraspinatous tendinitis
- tension neck syndrome
- thoracic outlet syndrome.

Tenosynovitis – A Case Of Mistaken Identity

In an occupational context a number of these conditions assume more importance than others. They are:-

- carpal tunnel syndrome
- de Quervain's disease
- Dupuytren's contracture
- tenosynovitis
- epicondylitis.

It is stressed that some conditions are not occupational in origin. There are also many other hand and arm disorders that do not have an occupational basis.

The cause of upper limb disorder is not solely physical – viral or bacterial infection and hormonal changes are also sometimes implicated.

Competing causes should always be explored and, where appropriate, given equal weight.

Hand And Wrist

Carpal Tunnel Syndrome

Also known as median neuritis, median thenar neuritis, median palsy or median neuropathy.

The term nocturnal numbness may also be used as symptoms are frequently most acute during rest.

Compression of the median nerve in the carpal tunnel caused by a repeated deviation of the wrist from the natural position and sometimes by local trauma or vibration leading to pain is known as carpal tunnel syndrome.

The carpal tunnel is a channel in the bones of the wrist through which pass the tendons in their sheath, the blood vessels and the median nerve responsible in part for feeling and movement in the palm, thumb and fingers of the hand.

Where tendons pass under bone they are enveloped in a sheath for protection and freedom of movement. One of the places where the tendons are enveloped in a sheath is where they pass under the retinaculum. The retinaculum is a fibrous band across the wrist which

Type Of Complaint

holds the tendons in place.

There are two such structures:-

1. The extensor retinaculum on the back of the wrist.
2. The flexor retinaculum on the palm or front side of the wrist.

The carpal tunnel passes beneath the flexor retinaculum which forms one of its sides – its other boundaries are formed by the bones of the wrist.

Chronic inflammation of the tendons or tendon sheaths may result in constriction (compression) of the median nerve thus affecting the areas of the hand and fingers supplied by the median nerve. These areas may vary from person to person but the common pattern involves the thumb, index, middle and part of the ring finger with resulting pain, discomfort and numbness in the palm and fingers on the lateral side of the hand and wrist often with an inability to move the fingers. Aching is not characteristic of this condition.

NB The median nerve does not supply all digits.

Carpal tunnel syndrome by itself is not recognised as a prescribed occupational disease but it is well recognised that it may follow flexor tenosynovitis (the long finger flexors pass with the median nerve through the carpal tunnel) and as such benefit may be paid in respect of disability arising therefrom.

Where it can be proved that the syndrome is associated with the performance of certain manual tasks (such as those that require active finger flexion with the wrist flexed) such cases can be considered an occupational disease. However, carpal tunnel syndrome occurs frequently in the general population usually without any obvious cause.

In effect any condition which might increase the volume of the structures within the carpal canal would tend to compress the nerve and carpal tunnel syndrome is the most commonly reported nerve entrapment syndrome.

A recent study by the HSE in collaboration with the Robens Institute at the University of Surrey found that 1.2 per thousand of the working population suffer from carpal tunnel syndrome.

Tenosynovitis – A Case Of Mistaken Identity

The highest risk group for the development of idiopathic (of no known cause) carpal tunnel syndrome is females between the ages of 40 and 60 years. It is a common condition among middle aged housewives possibly related to activities such as housework.

Most medical opinion suggests however that there is no evidence to indicate a direct causal relationship between the development of this condition and the repetitive wrist movements associated with specific occupations (apart from certain instances where it may follow flexor tenosynovitis as already noted). It is not impossible that at the time of an acute episode of flexor tenosynovitis, general swelling in the region of the front of the wrist may make the difference between freedom and entrapment of the median nerve in a person who was on the verge of compression of the nerve in any event.

Carpal tunnel syndrome in the absence of flexor tenosynovitis should not be regarded as an occupational upper limb disorder.

Carpal tunnel syndrome may also occur secondary to generalised systemic disease or local pathology at the wrist. The aetiological factors associated with carpal tunnel syndrome in this situation include:-

1. A decreased cross sectional area of the carpal tunnel such as occurs in rheumatoid arthritis or past fracture.
2. Increased volume of the contents of the carpal tunnel as may occur in flexor tenosynovitis, fluid retention in pregnancy, diabetes and thyroid disorder.
3. Enlargement of the median nerve (rare).

It is well recognised that carpal tunnel syndrome can recur after an interval despite adequate surgery.

De Quervain's Disease

De Quervain's disease, recognised as a traumatically induced occupational disease, is a progressively disabling condition of the hand at the junction of the thumb and wrist with persistent pain at the base of the thumb near the radial styloid.

Technically this condition is a stenosing tenosynovitis of the abductor pollicis longus and extensor pollicis brevis tendons of the thumb, a

Type Of Complaint

condition of thickening of the tendon sheath of the extensor and abductor muscle of the thumb with some impairment of free movement of these tendons.

Stenosis refers to a progressive restriction of the tendon sheath. Movement of the tendons becomes impossible resulting in partial incapacity of the thumb with constant and severe pain in the region of the radial styloid. Other features that may be present include radiation of pain down the thumb or up the forearm, weakness of the thumb, diminution of grip, tenderness and swelling over the tendon sheath and increased pain on wrist motion.

Pain is the predominant symptom. Crepitation is not a distinguishing feature.

The condition was described fully by de Quervain in 1895 and frequently bears his name (though he was not the first to describe it).

It is generally recognised that chronic trauma often in the form of prolonged exertion, repeated strain or unaccustomed muscular effort is the precipitating factor. Those manual workers engaged in ulnar deviation of the wrist combined with abduction of the thumb under the stress of a grasping or pinching motion are the likely candidates.

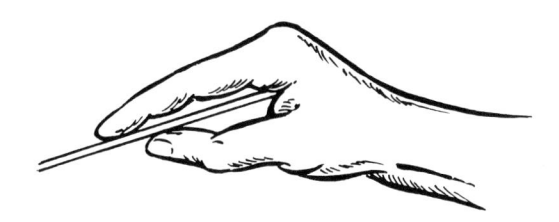

PULP PINCH

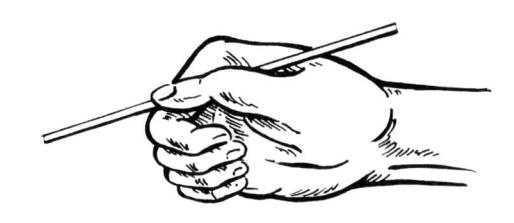

LATERAL PINCH

TENOSYNOVITIS – A CASE OF MISTAKEN IDENTITY

Trauma may not act alone. There is often an association with a predisposing constitutional factor. To that extent the condition can arise spontaneously. It is a common condition of the middle years predominantly among females in the 5th and 6th decades usually affecting the dominant hand and more commonly related to a single strain episode possibly associated with an inherent tendency to rheumatic condition.

The condition can become chronic. Chronicity implies that the inflamed sheaths around the involved tendons become narrow or stenosed. This is referred to as stenosing tenosynovitis.

In many cases surgery may be necessary to produce the desired relief.

Dupuytren's Contracture

This is a thickening and shortening of the palmar fascia – a fibrous fan in the palm of the hand which causes gradual and permanent bending of the fingers. The condition takes its name from a French surgeon who described it in 1832 but contracture of the tissues below the palm of the hand was known some two hundred years earlier.

It is a rare condition under the age of 40 years but much more common over the age of 60 years. The ring and little fingers are most often affected. Dupuytren's contracture occurs almost exclusively in people of European descent – it is virtually unknown in other races.

The cause of such condition is unknown but the disease is often inherited and there is an association with epilepsy, alcohol-related liver disease, chronic invalidism and tuberculosis. The role of occupation is much more dubious.

Many studies of the condition have revealed that it occurs equally in manual and non-manual workers and there is no definite causal relationship with occupation except perhaps to accelerate its appearance. There is however an alternative medical view that the development of the condition may be a sequel of repeated minor trauma to the palms of the hands. Such trauma can arise for example from heavy manual labour, from handling vibratory tools and from specific injury.

Contracture deformity develops insidiously and is usually neither painful nor disabling. Thus the amount of handicap varies and depends on occupation and attitude.

Treatment in the early stages is by means of exercise but the only cure is surgery to divide the fibrous bands beneath the skin.

Gamekeepers' Thumb

A stenosing condition of the thumb due to repeated abduction – extension force.

Ganglion

An enlargement on the sheath of a tendon or round a joint forming a swelling containing fluid most often on the back of the wrist. The cause of such swellings is unknown but is thought to be either some irregular growth of the synovial membrane and its secreting lubricating fluid or damage to the membrane following injury.

It is allegedly common in jobs with repeated wrist movement and may account for weakness in the wrist apart from cosmetic inconvenience. Treatment is simple and consists of encouraging absorption of the fluid by an injection or excision. Recurrence is common.

__Traditionally it is related that the cystic swelling was put under tension by flexing the wrist and the swelling hit with the family bible – a form of faith healing one assumes – the object being to rupture the cyst and release the fluid into the tissues where it would be absorbed.__

Tenosynovitis – A Case Of Mistaken Identity

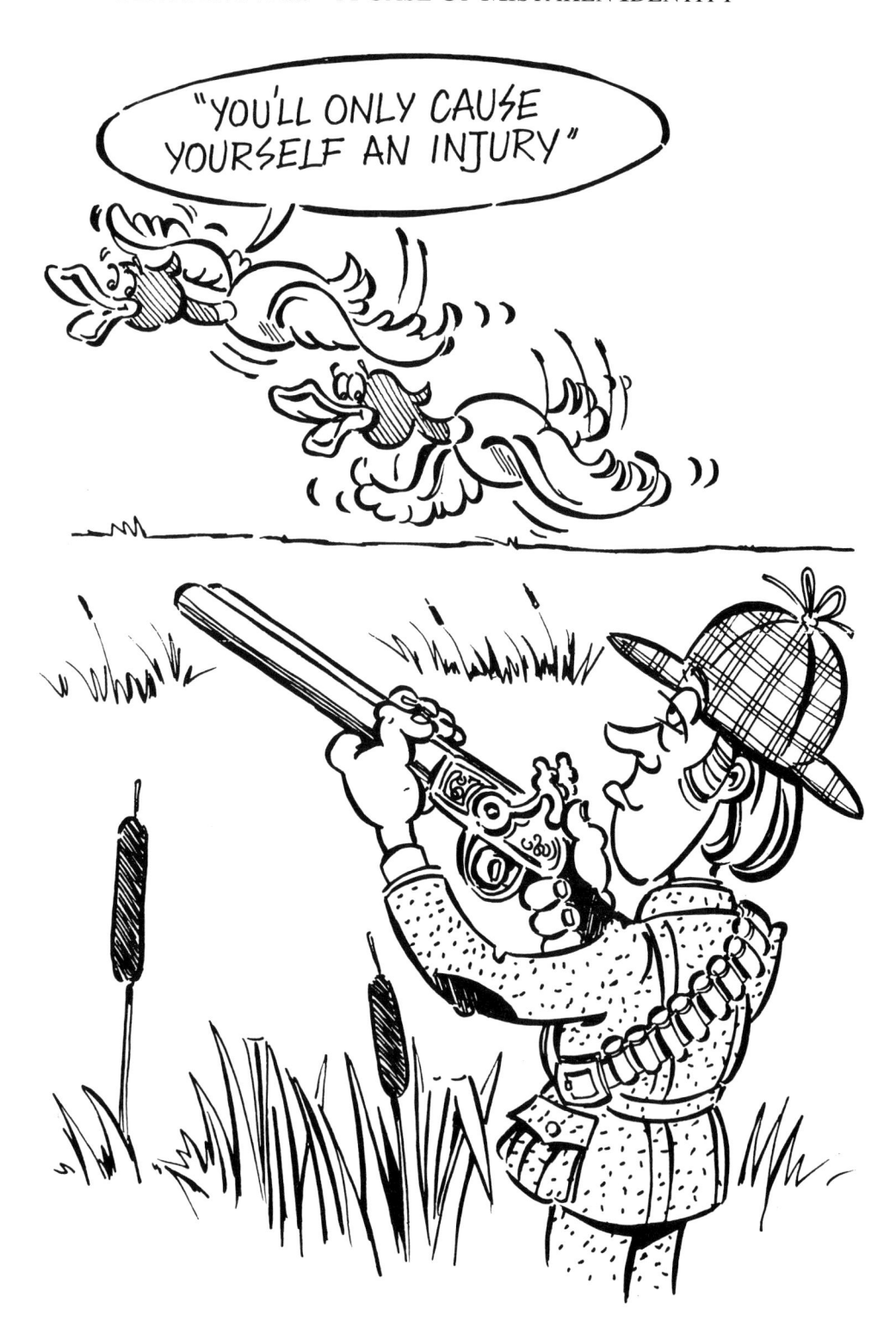

Type Of Complaint

Occupational Cramp

Cramp of the hand or forearm due to repetitive movement has been a prescribed disease in the form of telegraphists' cramp, writers' cramp and twisters' cramp since the early part of this century. Benefit can now be obtained for **any** type of occupational cramp arising from **manual activity** not necessarily from the previous specific occupations.

Occupational cramp is characterised by attacks of spasm, tremor and pain in the hand or forearm usually following some form of repeated muscular action. A continuing repetitive action will eventually result in loss of muscle co-ordination and an inability to perform fine repetitive movement.

At one time it was felt that the condition was purely a psychological one but the factors causative of the condition are unknown. Research has been unable to demonstrate any structural change in the central nervous system, the peripheral nerves or the muscles and the true cause is probably a combination of physical fatigue of muscles and nerves together with an underlying psychoneurosis.

Occupational cramp is a relatively rare condition that develops as a complicated reaction usually in operators concerned with skilled but repetitive tasks – possibly under stress and perhaps in a less than ideal environment.

The prognosis can be doubtful. The condition does not often respond to psychological treatment.

An entirely different form of cramp may affect those employees who undertake heavy physical work in high temperatures. Workers such as stokers, miners, foundry and rolling mill workers are the most likely to be affected. The cause is known to be salt depletion owing to excessive sweating and severe cases are rare. Onset is frequently sudden, usually in the later part of a working shift when pains may be experienced in the legs, arms, abdomen or back. Rest and saline drinks will usually effect a cure within a short time.

Tenosynovitis – A Case Of Mistaken Identity

Tenosynovitis

Traumatic inflammation of the tendons of the hand and forearm or of the associated tendon sheath is known as:-

1. **Peritendinitis crepitans** when the site of the lesion is in the tendons above the upper limit of the tendon sheath;
2. **Tenosynovitis** when the synovial lining of the tendon sheath is involved.

Tenosynovitis is a non-infective inflammatory reaction of the synovial sheath of the tendons, commonly in the hand, wrist and arm caused by unaccustomed and arduous exercise of the muscles of the forearm. This reaction may be present in either the flexor or extensor tendons giving rise to either **flexor tenosynovitis** or **extensor tenosynovitis**. Of the two the latter, involving the tendons on the back of the wrist and forearm, is the more common.

The tendons are enveloped by a tendon sheath the purpose of which is to provide lubrication when the tendon is passing under ligaments or round corners or in other positions where it needs this form of protection. Where free movement of a tendon is restricted within its sheath, the characteristic result is swelling of the radial aspect of the dorsum of the forearm, aching, pain and tenderness. In the early stages the subject may complain of a sore wrist and forearm – in the later stages the pain may be acute and movement of the wrist and fingers restricted.

Pressure on the tendon sheath will be painful and the ability to grip is lost. The pain can spread to the neck and shoulders. Crepitus may also be felt over the affected tendons. In advanced stages only jerky movement of the fingers may be possible and in the final stage the thumb or fingers may become locked in flexion.

Whilst any tendon may be involved, in industry it is the tendons of the hand, wrist and forearm that are more frequently affected. True tenosynovitis affects the tendon sheaths themselves, usually the extensors of the fingers.

Traumatic tenosynovitis is a frequent cause of incapacity in various occupations. It is commonly associated with any repetitive hand and arm activity in which frequent gripping or twist movements are required,

Type Of Complaint

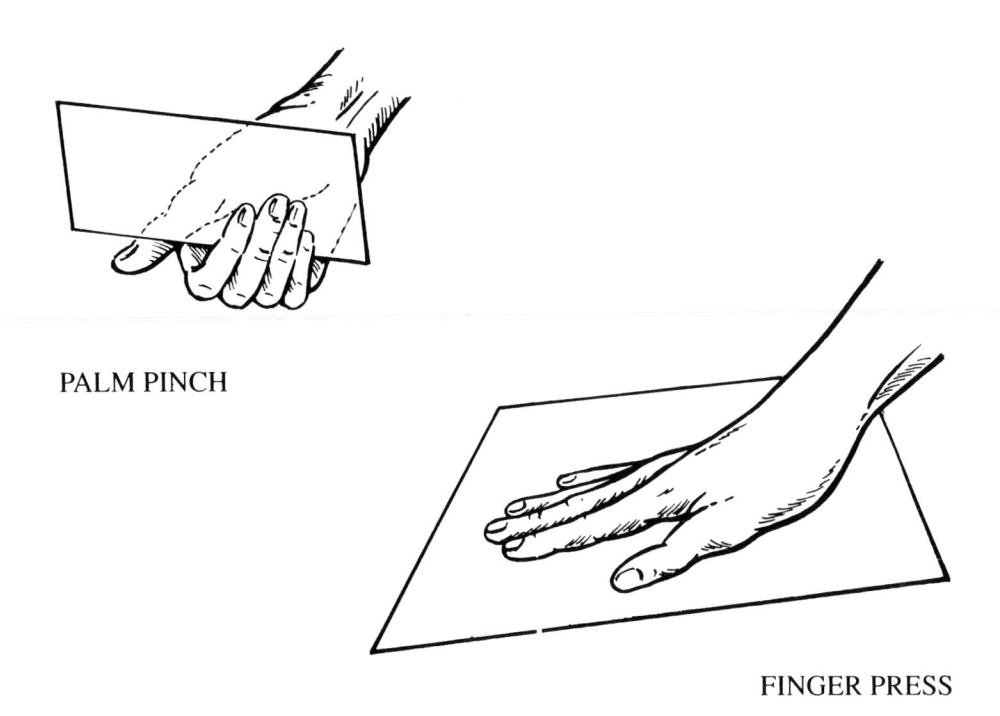

PALM PINCH

FINGER PRESS

especially those which involve a grasp between thumb and fingers accompanied by quick pronation/supination movement of the forearm. If the movements are made against resistance the risk is increased.

It is often caused by over-use but susceptibility is relevant.

Employees who have recently returned from holiday or sick leave are particularly vulnerable as are newcomers to repetitive jobs.

True tenosynovitis (as against the more common peritendinitis crepitans) is a comparatively rare condition.

Trigger Finger and Thumb (Stenosing Tenosynovitis Crepitans)

Trigger finger and thumb are due to a narrowing of the sheath of the flexor tendon at the level of the metacarpal neck, a nodular swelling of the tendon or both. The thumb is the digit most frequently involved – the index finger usually the least.

The condition occurs mostly in the female population in the ratio of about 4 to 1 and is predominant in the 5th and 6th decades. The finger becomes difficult to straighten after bending as free passage of the tendons becomes obstructed. As the tendon passes the site of the obstruction, a click or snap is often produced at the level of the metacarpal head where a reinforcement of deep fascia forms the proximal annular ligament or pulley in the sheath of the flexor tendon.

The cause of trigger finger and thumb is an excessive flexion or extension of the digits (or over-use) often associated with using tools that have handles with hard or sharp edges. If the annular ligament is pressed against the tendon by a hard object such as the handles of scissors, pruning shears or pliers, repeated movements of the fingers or thumb may cause irritation. In turn this irritation causes exudation and thickening of the tendon sheath and tendons just above and at the level of the sheath with effusion into the sheath.

As the condition becomes more marked, locking occurs and the tendon cannot move through the sheath without assistance.

The extensors are less strong than the flexors and normally locking takes place when the finger is flexed. The patient often demonstrates impaired extension or a temporary flexion deformity. Pain is not a feature.

If the condition does not respond to treatment such as hydrocortisone injection, then surgical excision of the constriction may be necessary.

Forearm And Elbow

Epicondylitis

The term epicondylitis means inflammation of the epicondyle of the elbow and occurs where the muscles join the bone at the elbow causing pain, swelling and discomfort.

Lateral epicondylitis, more commonly known as tennis elbow, describes a condition in which pain occurs as a result of inflammatory process localised to the lateral epicondyle of the humerus which is the site of origin of the extensor muscles of the wrist and fingers. It is a much more common complaint than medial epicondylitis or golfers elbow – this condition results from inflammation of the flexor muscle origin, the flexor muscles of the wrist and fingers arising from the medial epicondyle on the opposite side from the lateral epicondyle.

Type Of Complaint

These sporting names imply that there are risk factors other than occupation and the causal relationship between occupation and the condition is speculative.

The distinction may be important in cases allegedly arising from occupation.

The underlying pathology is however debatable.

Occupationally such a condition might occur in susceptible individuals when the arm is used for strong gripping and lifting. Common occupational risk factors are the use of heavy implements such as hammers, repeated supination and pronation of the forearm and forceful wrist extension movements. There are however many possible causes of this condition and sometimes no ascertained cause at all – it is a condition that can and does occur spontaneously. For instance the condition is very common in middle age – this is thought to be due to the natural or inevitable ageing process of wear and tear – where enthusiasm outruns the capacity of ageing joints.

One plausible theory is that the initiation of the epicondylitis requires a particular incident of strain of the muscles. Such a strain may not necessarily be very great and can occur from many causes but requires a movement which is uncommon in the everyday domestic situation and more when the elbow is constrained in its movements by the position required either in the workplace or by sporting activity.

Although common, the condition is transient. However, where there is denial of rest together with an impaired or poor healing tendency continued repetitive forearm use may cause the condition to become chronic. In this situation the demands of work could play a role in aggravating or exacerbating a minor complaint howsoever caused. With adequate treatment (in the form of enforced rest permitting healing) there is no reason why normality should not be returned. Injections of cortisone may be helpful in some cases.

A condition of epicondylitis due to over-use should normally recover following adequate treatment within 6 months. Any complaint remaining thereafter can reasonably be attributed to the presence of muscular and arthritic changes that develop gradually over the patient's lifetime.

It is for this reason that epicondylitis is such a common condition.

TENOSYNOVITIS – A CASE OF MISTAKEN IDENTITY

Peritendinitis Crepitans

Where the site of a lesion is in the tendons **above** the upper limit of the tendon sheath of the wrist the condition is known as **peritendinitis crepitans** and pathologically can be distinguished from the form of wrist lesion known as tenosynovitis which is a condition of the tendon **sheath**.

This lesion is much more common than a true tenosynovitis and generally regarded as more benign.

A long time ago it was given the name **Cellulite Peritendineuse** by the French medical specialist, Boyer.

The condition is characterised by localised swelling, pain and discomfort often accompanied by redness, local heat and sometimes (but not always) crepitus along the affected tendon or group of tendons and may be aggravated by pressure of movement.

Classically the patient develops a tender swelling some 4-12 cm proximal to the radial styloid on the back of the forearm at or near the musculo-tendinous junction where the radial wrist extensors cross under the abductor pollicis longus and extensor pollicis brevis muscles. The radial extensors of the wrist and abductors and extensors of the thumb are more frequently involved, sometimes alone but often in combination.

This is not a true tenosynovitis since the swelling, tenderness, pain (and perhaps crepitation) lie well above the upper limit of the **tendon sheath**.

Since Velpeau first observed tenosynovitis in 1818 it has widely been believed that the condition arises through fatigue and exhaustion of definite muscle groups resulting from unaccustomed work and over-exertion.

Howard in his 1937 paper concludes:-

1. Peritendinitis crepitans is the result of exhaustion of particular muscle groups by unaccustomed and unremitting toil or by continued, usual, accustomed labour following direct trauma.
2. The primary change is without doubt in the muscle, the other factors developing secondary to muscle exhaustion.
3. Adequate, complete immobilisation of joints and portions of the extremity moved by the affected muscles and tendons is the logical and most effective treatment.

Type Of Complaint

The work of Thompson & Plewes in 1951 and on which much of the subsequent Guidance Note MS.10 appears to have been based concluded that the main causes of tenosynovitis (ie peritendinitis crepitans) were prolonged exertion after unaccustomed work, resumption of work following absence and local trauma. The presence of muscle fatigue was noted in all cases.

They described 5 main aetiological factors:-

1. Occupational change necessitating unaccustomed movement.
2. Resumption of work after absence.
3. Repetitive stereotyped movement.
4. Direct local trauma.
5. Local "strain".

They suggest that "tenosynovitis" applied to the usual crepitating condition found proximal to the wrist joint is a misnomer. The actual site of the lesion is well above the upper limit of the tendon sheaths at the wrist – peritendinitis crepitans is a more accurate description.

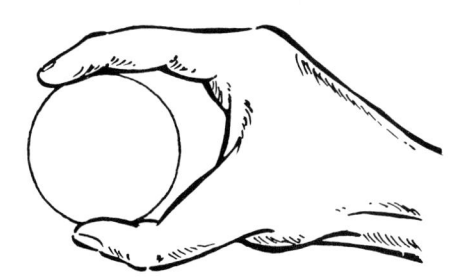

PULP GRASP

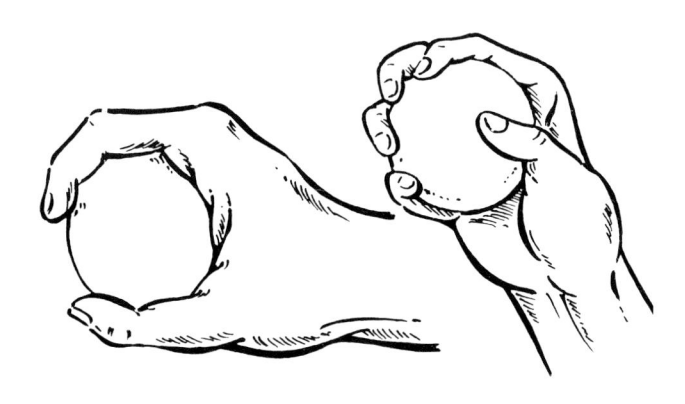

MEDIAL GRASP

Tenosynovitis – A Case Of Mistaken Identity

Pronator Teres Syndrome

Compression of the median nerve at the elbow as it passes through the two heads of the pronator teres (muscle) into the forearm. Found in occupations that involve rapid or resisted pronation and forceful pronation of the forearm with wrist flexion.

Radial Tunnel Syndrome

Peripheral entrapment of the radial nerve. May be caused by repeated rotary movements of the forearm with wrist flexion and extension.

Shoulder And Neck

Lesions in the shoulder and neck are common in work involving reaching or lifting and from the continuous use of the arm in abduction and flexion (in particular overhead work and carrying heavy objects) but may also have a non-occupational cause.

The most common shoulder tendon disorder is **rotator cuff tendinitis** or **supraspinatous tendinitis**. The wear and tear of repeated overhead motions contributes to the thickening of both tendons and bursae giving rise to the characteristic **frozen shoulder** syndrome causing pain and impaired function.

The shoulder is also a frequent target for degenerative joint disease and rheumatoid arthritis.

Thoracic outlet syndrome is a neurovascular disorder that involves the shoulder and upper arm. It may be regarded as a general term for compression of the nerves and blood vessels between the neck and arm. Symptoms, namely numbness and tingling in the fingers of the hand and arm, are similar to those of carpal tunnel syndrome.

NB   Spondylitis, inflammation of the synovial joints of the neck, is a common condition of the neck and spine rather than hand and arm.

CAUSE OF UPPER LIMB DISORDERS

Occupational Risk Factors

A risk factor is defined as an attribute or exposure that increases the probability of the disease or disorder.

Several principal risk factors can be identified but in the absence of any concrete evidence to link particular factors with specific health effects, the aetiology of upper limb disorder as with many other medical conditions should be considered as multifactorial in origin.

The causes of musculo-skeletal problems are multiple and complex but broadly risk factors fall into two groups:-

- biomechanical factors
- unsafe systems of work.

TENOSYNOVITIS – A CASE OF MISTAKEN IDENTITY

Biomechanical Factors

Repetition and Force — The degree of simple repetitive and/or forceful activity required.

Static Muscle Load — The task may involve working from a visibly awkward position such as to cause **physical stress.**

Bad Posture — Often not as visible or obvious but may also impose physical stress.

Mechanical Stress — Action beyond the degree of force exerted by the average human hand which may be accentuated by badly designed equipment.

Vibration — Which imposes greater hand force requirements eg from powered tools.

The Thermal Environment and Quality of Air — The effects of temperature, air quality and movement and humidity.

The Visual Environment — The effects of visual fatigue and ocular discomfort.

Noise — Though rarely anywhere near hearing damage levels, equipment noise can be annoying and disruptive especially to those performing tasks that require sustained concentration.

NB *It is the combined effect of those conditions and the personal preferences of occupants which determine whether an environment is judged to be satisfactory or not.*

Direct Local Trauma — Such as a knock or blow to a vulnerable area of the body.

Leisure & Household Activities — Sporting, leisure pursuits, hobbies as well as household duties are of particular relevance.

CAUSE OF UPPER LIMB DISORDERS

Unsafe Systems of Work

1. Work Rate

- the application of effort and speed
- organisation of work rate
- excessive demands
- shortage of labour
- peak demands
- pressure of work
- bonus/incentive/piecework systems
- compulsory overtime/excessive hours
- alteration to method or tempo of work
- rapid introduction/insufficient period of adjustment.

2. Lack of Task Variation

- difficulty of task
- repetition of task and boredom where no rotation is possible
- inadequate rest breaks and work pauses.

3. Poor Supervision

- lack of control over job
- failure to respond to complaints and/or other reports
- failure to monitor resumption of work following absence such as return from holiday or illness
- new labour
- change of occupation necessitating unaccustomed work.

4. The Working Area

- poor workplace, tool and equipment design
- poorly maintained equipment
- introduction of new tools.

Tenosynovitis – A Case Of Mistaken Identity

5. Delayed Symptom Reporting and Incorrect Diagnosis

- failure to instruct and warn.

6. Personnel Services

- inadequate training, rehabilitation and other personnel functions.

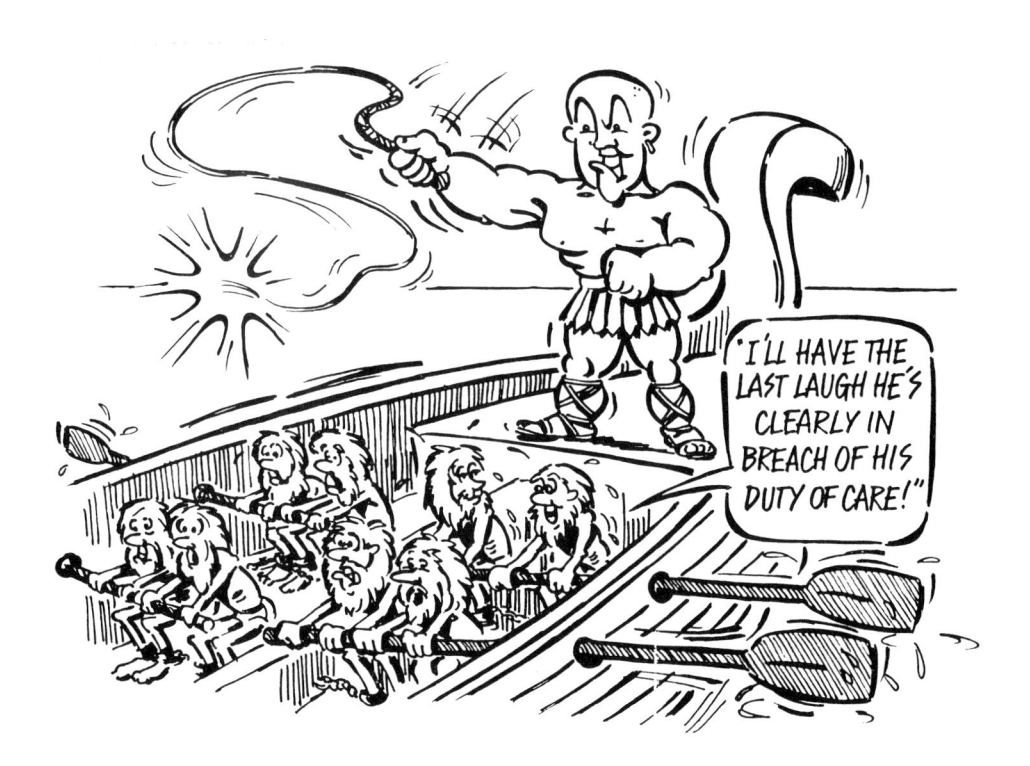

CONTROL & MANAGEMENT OF UPPER LIMB DISORDERS

Control and management of upper limb disorders may be considered under the specific headings of:-
- treatment
- prevention.

Treatment

Medical treatment lies in the accurate clinical assessment of patients complaining of occupational upper limb disorder and in differentiating the clearly defined physical conditions from non-physical and non-occupational sources. There is an element of susceptibility, and reaction to treatment will vary widely – clear advice from the outset is thus essential. Where specific treatment and encouragement is given most sufferers can be restored to a full range of pain free activity.

Treatment may take the form of one or more of the following remedies:-

- **Rest through cessation of occupation**

    Cessation of occupation is inevitable if the symptoms are severe and desirable where there is a risk that symptoms may progress from minor discomfort to a higher risk situation.

    Cure is frequently achieved by resting the limb concerned to allow the swollen tendon/tendon sheath to recover. The patient should refrain from the occupation or other activity causing the condition. If such occupation or activity is removed at the outset, early healing may take place. Conversely the demands of work or activity are likely to cause the condition to become chronic.

- **Immobilisation of affected part**

    Limiting movement by encasing in plaster may be a desirable remedy in severe cases.

    In persistent cases the following additional remedies may be relevant:-

- **Injection**

    Hydrocortisone injection is a common treatment but not always successful.

- **Physiotherapy**
- **Analgesics**
- **Anti-inflammatory drugs**
- **Anti-depressants**
- **Operation**

These additional remedies are in a more doubtful category of treatment.

A gradual reintroduction to work combined with health monitoring is likely to have the greatest chance of success.

Prevention & Risk Reduction

Often the most effective way of dealing with occupational upper limb disorder is through preventative strategies at the workplace.

Preventative measures may be grouped under one or more of the following headings but in view of large personal variations in susceptibility as well as other medical and non-medical factors they may not apply precisely to every situation:-

- engineering controls and ergonomic factors
- organisation of works systems
- competent personnel function
- knowledge and warning
- risk assessment and planning.

CONTROL & MANAGEMENT

1. Engineering Controls and Ergonomic Factors

Engineering Controls means the physical measures that can be taken to eliminate or minimise repetitive movement by automation within the workplace or alternatively redesign, modification or adjustment of the tools used.

Ergonomics is derived from the Greek **ergon** meaning **work** and **nomos** meaning **law** but is not a discipline that can be traced back to ancient times.

The human frame is both adaptable and flexible in a wide range of activities. In the past this adaptability has allowed humans to tolerate a working environment that frequently was ill-suited to their requirements, often to their psychological and physical detriment.

The idea behind the concept of ergonomics is that of matching equipment and machinery to the individual and the working environment – "the fit between people, the equipment they use and the environment they work in" as described by one commentator.

The modern origins of the discipline may be found in the Second World War where it became a necessity for inexperienced armed services personnel to handle sophisticated machinery with the minimum of training.

At that time ergonomics was defined as:-

> "the study, by physiological and psychological methods, of the best means of increasing the operational efficiency, safety and comfort of soldiers, sailors and aviators under different environmental conditions and, conversely, the adaptation of ships, fighting vehicles, aircraft and weapons to the convenience of those who have to use them".

The subsequent application of the definition to the workplace was a logical step.

The modern ergonomic approach to workplace design is based on the factors that influence the observed relationship and effectiveness of individual and machine. Such factors must be determined by a systematic and scientific analysis of the system of work as a whole and those individuals who contribute towards it.

Under this general heading the following topics need to be considered:-

Workplace Design – in general the area designated to the allotted task should be designed to provide:-

Tenosynovitis – A Case Of Mistaken Identity

- sufficient working space to enable the operator to work in comparative comfort and safety without excessive twisting, turning or arm elevation
- reasonable movement within the working area where required
- adequate access to and from the various component parts of the job.

Equipment Design – where practicable the replacement or modification of old or poorly designed equipment should have a high priority.

Examples of poorly designed equipment are numerous – tools that are too large, too small or simply improvised – tools with a jerky or inconsistent action – equipment requiring a great deal of effort to operate and maintain in operation – poor handle design.

The workstation itself is often a source of potential hazard – where practicable adjustable equipment should be supplied.

The main aim of the adjustable workstation is to eliminate operator stress and fatigue. However, the availability of adjustable equipment per se does not necessarily provide the solution. The purchase and use of adjustable equipment needs to be combined with appropriate education and training.

Posture and Mechanical Stress – whilst mental stress may be a feature of susceptibility, physical or mechanical stress is closely related to posture and can often be eliminated by the relatively simple measure of redesigning or adjusting the equipment or tooling enabling the operator to work with a much higher degree of comfort. Examples of this are height (of a workbench) – seating – position of the feet – elevation of the forearm. Operators rarely have a uniform height and shape. The aim wherever possible should be to eliminate any physical tension that is likely to be present.

The Thermal Environment – thermal comfort is a complex area in which it is impossible to satisfy everyone's requirements all the time. Human thermal comfort is influenced by six major factors:-

- metabolic work rate
- clothing worn
- air temperature
- relative humidity
- air movement
- radiant heat loss or gain.

CONTROL & MANAGEMENT

"OPERATORS RARELY HAVE A UNIFORM HEIGHT AND SHAPE"

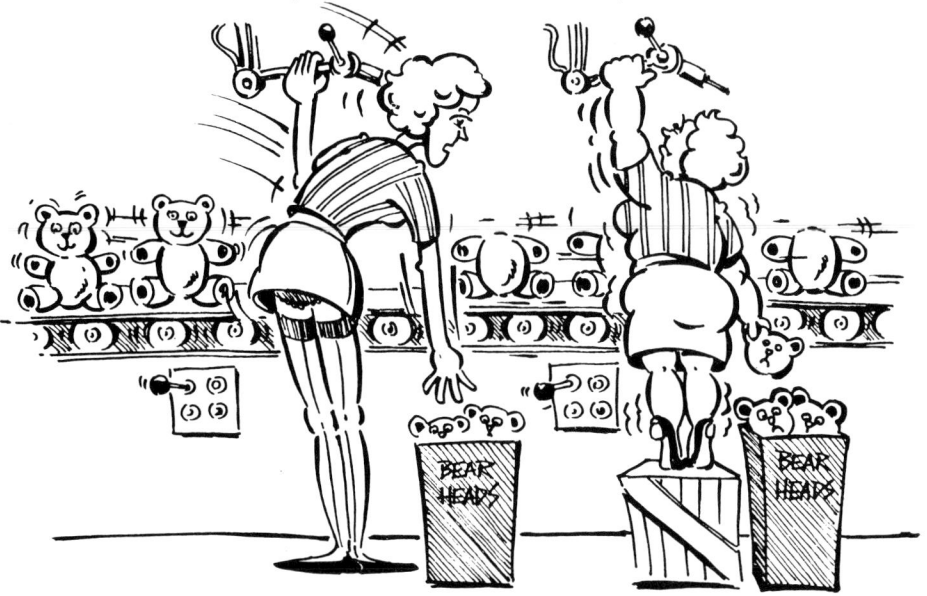

Over-warm conditions are as uncomfortable as cold conditions. The aim should be to achieve a balanced temperature.

The Visual Environment – Three factors are relevant:-

- lighting
- visual task required
- eyesight of operator.

Visual requirements can influence the posture adopted by the user. Thus visual tasks may be a contributory factor not only to visual fatigue but also to musculo-skeletal discomfort. It is therefore important not only to have adequate or appropriately corrected eyesight but also adequately designed workstations.

Vibration – Elimination or reduction of excessive vibration by, for example, the provision of ergonomically designed tooling to minimise hand force requirements is desirable. Vibration at particular frequencies is associated with vascular and neurological problems and could affect muscle and tendon blood supply exacerbating force and motion problems.

The overall aim should be to determine the vulnerable elements of the job

Tenosynovitis – A Case Of Mistaken Identity

(or alternatively to isolate the vulnerable person). To that end, a job survey or ergonomic study should be implemented if any risk is suspected or foreseen. This may involve investigating all complaints and recording every factor relating to workstation location and layout.

2. Organisation of Works Systems

Many production line operations and techniques are repetitive and boring but as they are frequently well paid, such operations are tolerated. Due to wide variations in susceptibility some individuals may have shorter tolerance times than others but which individuals are vulnerable is not easy to determine.

Attention should therefore be directed initially towards the modification of work processes to minimise such activities as forcible movement of the thumb, pronation/supination of the wrist, flexion/extension of the wrist and rotation of the shoulder with the arm elevated. Some obvious questions are:-

- Can the job be slowed down without loss of efficiency or output?
- Are bonus systems and piecework rates necessary?
- Are there sufficient natural breaks?
- Is rationing of tasks possible?

In the type of operation with which this complaint is concerned, it is advisable to use natural breaks to their fullest advantage.

For example with a Visual Display Unit operation it is desirable that the maximum **continuous** use should be restricted in duration. In an unpublished study by Professor Tom Cox of Nottingham University commissioned by the Health and Safety Executive it was recommended that the maximum acceptable time of exposure to repetitive VDU work without a break is around 120 minutes and the desirable time without a break around 50-60 minutes. Research indicated that accuracy fell over extended work periods of two to three hours. After 50-60 minutes of working the break needed to be around 12-15 minutes to have any significant beneficial effect on mood and performance.

There is some variance from this advice in the guidance issued by the Health & Safety Executive with the introduction of The Health & Safety (Display Screen Equipment) Regulations 1992. They suggest short, frequent breaks are more satisfactory than occasional, longer breaks. Thus a break of 5-10 minutes

CONTROL & MANAGEMENT

after continuous working of 50-60 minutes is likely to be more beneficial than a 15 minute break every two hours.

Some people may prefer more frequent but shorter breaks.

Rest pauses should be introduced to prevent tiredness. They should be taken prior to the onset of fatigue, not to recuperate from it. Natural breaks resulting in reduction of muscle tension are greatly assisted by a system of job rotation where possible. However job rotation can require a great deal of additional training and management and does not remove the causes of strain. Guidance on rest cannot be specific since it is likely that if strict mandatory rest times are enforced, they may often be found to be unnecessarily prolonged and frustrating for some and for others too short to prevent the onset of fatigue.

3. Competent Personnel Function

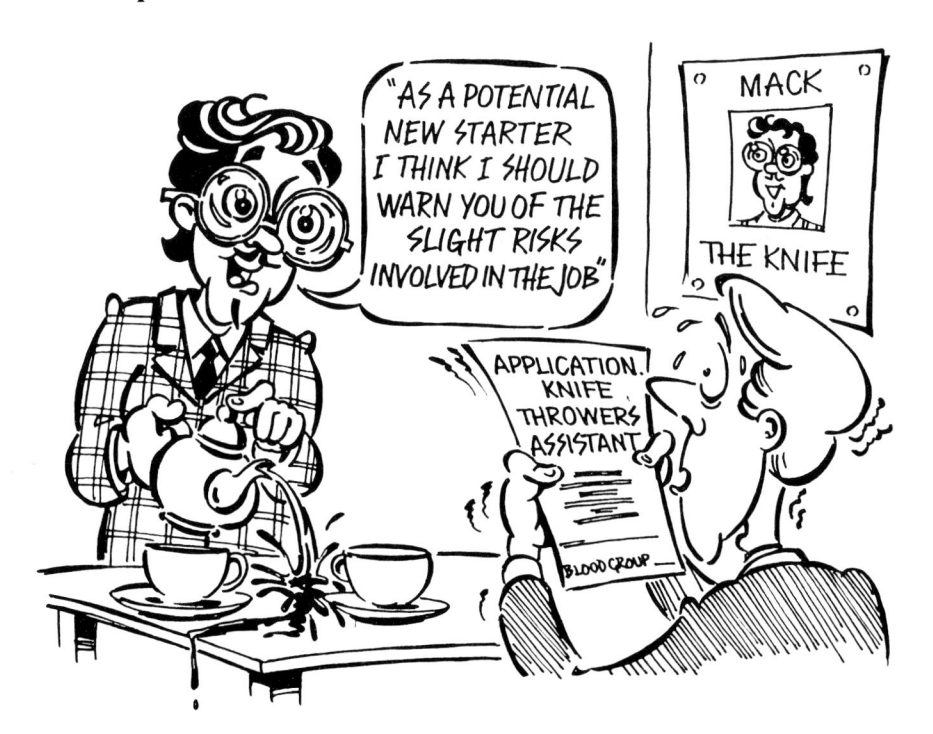

Pre-employment Interview – Should be conducted by a responsible person and involve the use of a pre-employment questionnaire. This should direct questions to pre-existing health problems. Where risk of injury is within the knowledge of the potential employer, new starters should be alerted. In such circumstances any offer of employment should contain a suitable warning of the risks involved and an opportunity given to accept or reject the offer of employment. Whilst there is no obligation, a warning along these lines is advisable.

Early Symptom Reporting – Most successful prevention campaigns have been directed towards encouraging employees to report symptoms early. This assumes knowledge by the employer – constructive or actual – of the potential problem. It is important that the symptoms are diagnosed at an early stage whilst the condition is still reversible. The kind of symptoms that may arise and the problems likely to cause them should be stressed. These include tiredness, fatigue and any unusual aches affecting the arms, hand and wrist. Such symptoms may appear trivial but reporting enables early investigation to be undertaken. Reports may be made either to the employer direct or to the patient's General Practitioner.

Action Taken – **Prompt** action **must** be taken once the employer is aware of the situation. Knowledge may arise either from an actual case report or from complaints from the workforce. Complaints should not be ignored – management must be shown to have taken positive action. Appropriate action includes:-

- referral to patient's own GP
- referral to works doctor
- Personnel Department counselling
- consideration of alternative employment (if available)

NB *Alternative employment frequently pays less;*

- advice to rest.

Advice to cease work completely may not necessarily be the best course of action to follow unless there is a known history of complaint, nor a change of employment at the time of the first report as the condition could settle of its own accord. Repetitive work could however prolong the condition and the employer must be alert to continuing symptoms.

Monitoring and Periodical Review – Where medical advice is given to the effect that cessation or change of occupation is unnecessary, the employer may take a conscious decision to allow the employee to continue working at the same repetitive task. In such circumstances it is imperative that the work done following this decision is fully monitored and periodically reviewed. Monitoring and review is a personnel function but could be delegated to some other competent person such as a safety officer.

The movement initially involved should be re-introduced only gradually – a realistic approach for which employers should not be criticised. This may involve temporary change in activities for a few days or a few weeks at the most.

A system of monitoring should also include:-

- review of the Accident Book on a regular basis
- liaison with the company doctor and medical centre/first aider/nurse
- observation and review of new starters and those employees at risk upon:-
    - return from holiday
    - assignment of new task
    - introduction of new process
    - increase in the rate of work
- discussion with union representative.

Training – The level and depth of training may have an important bearing on the incidence of upper limb disorder. Powers of concentration, co-ordination and relaxation must be taught alongside practical task training to ensure that an operator achieves the correct level of skill and strength required to achieve maximum efficiency.

A systematic approach to training should form part of the Company Health and Safety policy. Training may take the form of either **pre-employment** (or **induction**) training or **on the job** training and assumes importance in upper limb disorder cases as it provides an ideal opportunity to stress the minimal risks involved and the importance of early symptom reporting. The best ergonomically designed workstation will confer little benefit if the operator has not been adequately trained in its use.

4. Knowledge and Warning

Employers frequently ask whether there is a duty to warn, being mindful that alarm may be caused by doing so. On the other hand in a litigation scenario the plaintiff's case often lays great stress on the **duty to warn** without specifying precisely what form such warning should take.

Two kinds of warning may be relevant:-

- pre-employment
- early symptom reporting.

Awareness, knowledge and foreseeability on the part of the employer are implicit.

A **pre-employment** warning may take the form of fully counselling and advising the **prospective** employee of the repetitive (and usually forceful) nature of the work or process that is to be undertaken and of possible reaction or risk of injury that may occur given that all individuals are different and have varying degrees of susceptibility.

At the outset therefore the prospective employee must consider as a condition of employment whether or not to accept whatever minimal risks may be present, that is minimal risk of a minimal occurrence or degree of discomfort or injury.

If, despite the warning of minimal risks, the offer of employment is accepted and a disorder of the upper limb contracted, the employer should not be liable. The duty however is a continuous, one more, especially where the nature of the work changes possibly to a heavier and more demanding job. Guidance can be gained from case law:-

In **PRESLAND -v- PADLEY** it was held that an employer is under a duty in cases where the nature of the work carries an inherent, specific and not insignificant risk of a servant developing an industrial disease or condition to tell the servant at the beginning of the employment about the risk in order to allow the servant the option whether to embark on the employment or not.

In **PEPALL & OTHERS -v- THORN** the court found that whilst there was no duty on this **particular employer** to warn **prospective** employees of the risk of tenosynovitis (or related condition) because at that stage, which was prior to training, it would not be known what work a given employee would be doing, nevertheless there was a duty upon the employer to warn and **to continue**

to warn when a person was put on work that involved an inherent, specific and not insignificant risk of developing tenosynovitis or a similar condition (following **PRESLAND -v- PADLEY**).

In **WHITE -v- HOLBROOK PRECISION CASTINGS** (a vibration white finger case) the Court of Appeal in upholding the decision of the judge at first instance came to the following conclusion. "What should an employer tell a prospective employee about the risks he will expose himself to if he takes the job? Generally speaking if the job has risks to health and safety which are not common knowledge, but of which an employer knows or ought to know and against which he cannot guard by taking precautions, then he should tell anyone to whom he is offering the job what those risks are if, from the information then available to him, knowledge of those risks would be likely to affect the decision of a sensible, level-headed prospective employee about accepting the offer".

Once the sensible, level-headed employee has accepted the offer of employment on those terms the employer is subsequently under no legal duty to **dismiss** the employee who wishes to continue working even though the employer is **aware** of some slight risk to the employee.

In **WITHERS -v- PERRY CHAIN** (a dermatitis case) the Court of Appeal held that employers were under no duty to dismiss or refuse to employ an adult employee who wished to do a job merely because there might be some **slight** risk to the employee in doing the work.

Some assistance is also derived from the cases of **JOSEPH -v- MINISTRY OF DEFENCE** (a vibration white finger case) and **LANE -v- SUN VALLEY POULTRY** (a tenosynovitis case).

Given that the employee has elected to continue working, the second leg of the warning, that of **early symptom reporting,** does however take on considerable significance. Those decisions in the courts which have gone against the employers are frequently based on factors of warning and early symptom reporting. The risk here is that of permanent disablement if the work continues and no action is taken. The warning must be specific.

This duty must logically extend to the existing workforce.

In **BURGESS -v- THORN** it was held that it would have been simple to have warned the workforce that if they started having pain in the wrist or arm, they must report it at once and consult their doctor because it might indicate the presence of a condition which, if dealt with promptly would be innocuous but if not dealt with might soon become serious enough to require surgery.

Dependence upon the employee reporting complaints may not always meet the requirements of an adequate system of early symptom reporting. In **PEPALL & OTHERS -v- THORN** it was held that what was required was a process of **regular** education bringing home to the employee the particular steps that could be taken having regard to the nature of the work.

5. Risk Assessment and Planning

As part of a preventative strategy, a formal policy on upper limb disorder should be established and employees made aware of its existence. Where a particular job or range of jobs is suspect, some form of risk assessment should be made to identify the specific risk factors. Where risk assessment is likely to be complex, expert help should be sought.

The object of any risk assessment programme should be to create a better working environment, to fulfil legal obligations to the workforce and to prevent potentially expensive claims. Such a programme would need to be developed to suit the individual needs of the company and to involve the co-operation of not only the workforce, but of all levels of management. In broad outline the programme would need to incorporate the following measures:-

- an initial assessment
- a detailed survey report
- formulation and implementation of a long term plan to reduce awkward working postures
- education and training
- formal reporting and auditing systems.

Well designed tasks will show the following characteristics:-
- **variety** in the activities and skills used
- a degree of **individual control** over the place of work
- some **cohesion** with the work of the organisation
- opportunity for the individual to use skills and experience
- sufficient feedback on quality and quantity of task performance.

A good implementation plan will consider whether changes are necessary

Control & Management

in such areas as:-

- employee selection and placement
- training
- job content and career paths
- organisational structure
- system requirements
- personnel policies.

Of all the recommendations contained in this section it is considered that the most important, once the employer knows or ought to know of the possibility of injury, is the warning to those potentially at risk. The warning should spell out what the job entails; that while everything has been done to obviate the risk some individuals may have a particular susceptibility to injury; that anyone starting to suffer aches and pains must report to the ambulance room, the nurse, the works doctor, the supervisor or should consult their own General Practitioner.

The warning may be contained in a notice in pay packets, in which event a record must be kept of when and to whom it is given. Alternatively it may be by a "teach in", in which event a record must be kept of what was said, by whom, and who attended.

Plain language is essential. Employers should be sure that the warning message has been understood. Once the employer has done all that is reasonably practicable to obviate the risk and appropriate warnings have been given, then should an individual present with complaints or symptoms it is for the employee to make an important decision. If alternative work is available it should be offered. If not, the employee should be told he has a personal susceptibility to strain injury. If he wants to seek alternative employment elsewhere so be it but if not he should be warned of the risk if he elects to work on. **An employee may accept a minimal risk of minimal injury.** The employer should not be at risk of liability in such circumstances.

What constitutes a "minimal risk" is a matter of judgement reached jointly, if possible, by the interested parties including the employee. What is important is to demonstrate that the degree of risk has been debated.

PRESCRIPTION AND OFFICIAL GUIDANCE

Prescription

Upper limb disorder in a very limited form has been a prescribed disease since **1907**. Prescription resulted from evidence placed in 1906 before the Departmental Committee on Compensation for Industrial Diseases. They considered the evidence under the heading **Sprained Wrist and Tenosynovitis** and concluded:-

> "Inflammation of the synovial lining of the wrist joint and tendon sheaths may occur among miners, not through accident, but through a long succession of jars to the wrist due to working a pick in hard coal".

Inclusion in the Schedule to the Workmen's Compensation Act 1906 was subsequently recommended by the report of the Committee issued in 1907 (Command 3495) and thereafter appeared under the following description:-

> "Inflammation of the synovial lining of the wrist joint and tendon sheaths":-

a limited prescription applicable to **mining only.**

Between 1908 and 1922 the Schedule was extended to include the following hand/arm conditions:-

- telegraphists' cramp through the use of telegraphic instruments
- writers' cramp as a result of unspecified processes
- twisters' cramp caused by twisting of cotton or woollen (including worsted) yarns.

Prescription And Official Guidance

A person suffering from twisters' cramp was not entitled to compensation under the provisions of the section unless totally disabled from following the occupation of a twister.

A person suffering from writers' cramp was entitled to compensation under the provisions of the section on account of that condition for not more than 12 months.

The prescription for sprained wrist and tenosynovitis remained the same.

It was not until the National Insurance (Industrial Injuries) (Prescribed Diseases) Regulations came into operation on 30 June 1948 that prescription of hand and arm conditions was extended and widened in the following terms:-

PD.28 Telegraphists' Cramp

Nature of Occupation
The use of morse-key telegraphic instruments for prolonged periods.

PD.29 Writers' Cramp

Nature of Occupation
Hand writing for prolonged periods.

PD.30 Twisters' Cramp

Nature of Occupation
The twisting of cotton or woollen (including worsted) yarn.

PD.34 Inflammation of the Synovial Lining of the Wrist Joint and Tendon Sheaths

Nature of Occupation
Manual labour, or frequent or repeated movements of the hand or wrist.

In the 1950 edition of Notes on the Diagnosis of Occupational Diseases, **PD.34** (Inflammation of the synovial lining of the wrist joint and tendon sheaths) is described in the following terms:-

Aetiology
Synovitis in these situations is a non-infective condition brought about by sudden strain, by unaccustomed and arduous exercise of the forearm muscles, or by repeated jarring of the hand, wrist or forearm such as

occurs in using a pick against hard rock or coal. The parts affected are the tendon sheaths of the carpal canal and of the thumb extensor tendons. The traumatised synovial membrane becomes congested and exudes lymph, or there is a "friction rub". In its later stages, incomplete resolution may result in adhesions. The condition does not normally go on to suppuration, but existing tubercular infection may become localised in the area concerned when there is a chronic effusion with weakness and continued incapacity.

Diagnosis
The onset is usually sudden with loss of power in the arm and swelling of the forearm and wrist. Movement, at first painful and accompanied by a characteristic harsh rub, becomes limited as the effusion appears and increases.

Prognosis
The condition usually clears up completely with rest and conservative treatment but occasionally becomes chronic.

Since 1948 there have been two major changes in prescription. Both came about as a result of recommendations made in a report by the Industrial Injuries Advisory Council in April 1958 following a Review of the Prescribed Diseases Schedule. The recommendations were as follows:-

Telegraphists', Writers' & Twisters' Cramp (disease numbers 28, 29 and 30)

"It appears to us that the need is for a description of these disorders which would avoid reference to specific processes. Our recommendation is that the three cramps at present prescribed should be replaced by one description – **cramp of the hand or forearm due to repetitive movements.** The occupational cover recommended is – **any occupation involving prolonged periods of handwriting, typing or other repetitive movements of the fingers, hand or arm.** We consider this should cover the three forms of cramp at present prescribed as well as affording cover to typists, linotype operators and other workers whose work entails repetitive movements."

PRESCRIPTION AND OFFICIAL GUIDANCE

Inflammation of the Synovial Lining of the Wrist Joint & Tendon Sheaths (disease number 34)

"The description of this disease was criticised on two counts in the representations we received. The first was that in order to claim benefit for the disease it has to be shown that both the synovial lining of the wrist joint and the tendon sheaths are affected whereas in some cases which are undoubtedly of occupational origin, it may not be possible to demonstrate both conditions.

Secondly it was pointed out that the prescription is too restrictive in that it covers neither cases of inflammation of the tendon sheaths in the fingers and thumb, nor cases where the tendons themselves, and not their sheaths, are affected.

We agree that both these criticisms mentioned above which are at present omitted satisfy the requirements for prescription.

Essentially what the prescription should, in our opinion, cover is inflammation of either the tendons themselves in the hand or forearm or of the sheaths in which the tendons are enclosed. Where this condition is occupational in origin it is due to friction or repeated movements of the hand or the wrist, as is indicated in the present occupational cover.

We accordingly recommend that the disease be redefined as – **traumatic inflammation of the tendons of the hand or forearm, or of the associated tendon sheaths.**

The occupational cover should remain as at present – **any occupation involving manual labour, or frequent or repeated movements of the hand or wrist.**"

Tenosynovitis – A Case Of Mistaken Identity

Tennis Elbow

The prescription of tennis elbow was considered but rejected. It was found that on the evidence available there was no justification for ascribing an occupational origin to the condition. Clearly it would be essential to have some reliable information on the incidence of this disease in a variety of occupations before it would be possible to decide whether the conditions for prescription are satisfied.

Accordingly it was recommended that the Council should invite the Ministry to put in hand an inquiry into the incidence of elbow conditions in trades involving manual labour compared with other sections of the community. The Council specifically had bricklaying brought to their notice in this connection – particular attention should be given to this trade.

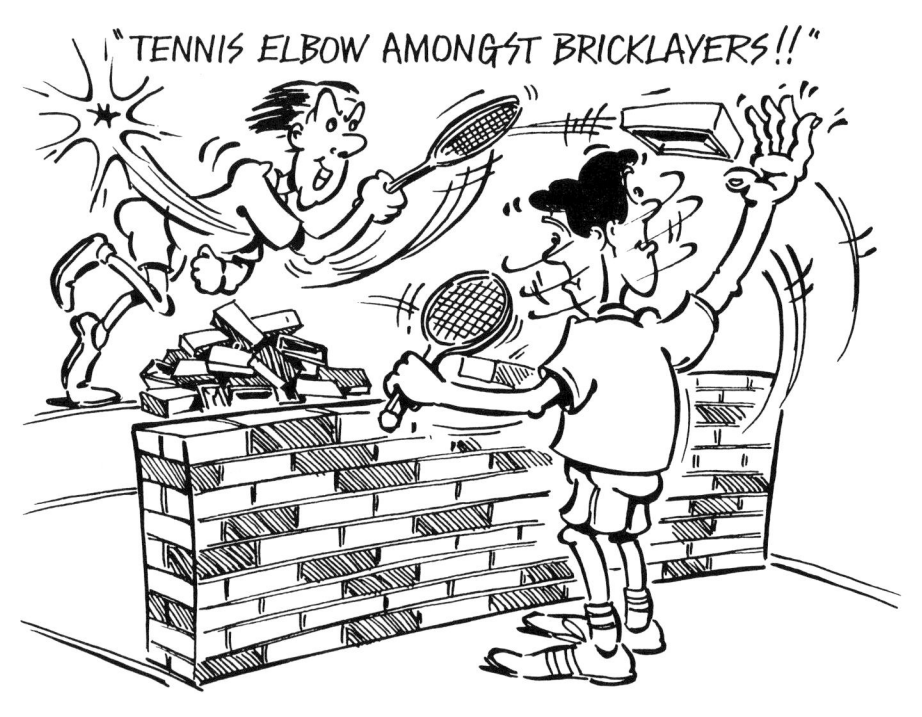

NB *At the present time tennis elbow is still not a prescribed disease.*

The recommendations were given formal legal status by the National Insurance (Industrial Injuries) (Prescribed Diseases) Amendment Regulations 1958 which came into effect on 7 July 1958.

PRESCRIPTION AND OFFICIAL GUIDANCE

The former separately prescribed diseases of PD.28, PD.29 and PD.30 namely telegraphists' cramp, writers' cramp and twisters' cramp are now all included in PD.28 under the description:-

PD.28 Cramp of the Hand or Forearm due to Repetitive Movements

Nature of Occupation
Prolonged periods of handwriting, typing or other repetitive movements of the fingers, hand or arm.

This became PD.A4 in 1983 when major changes were made to the Schedule of prescribed diseases. Notes on the Diagnosis of Occupational Diseases describe the condition as follows:-

Aetiology
This disability, known also as writers' cramp, telegraphists' cramp, twisters' cramp, occupational cramp, or craft palsy.......................... encompassing **not only** the previously described specific occupational conditions but now also **any** type of occupational cramp.

The other major change is that PD.34 (since 1983 – PD.A8) is now described as:-

PD.34 Traumatic Inflammation of the Tendons of the Hand or Forearm or of the Associated Tendon Sheaths

Nature of Occupation
Manual labour, or frequent or repeated movement of the hand or wrist thus widening the description still further.

Notes on the Diagnosis of Occupational Diseases describe the condition as follows:-

Aetiology
This condition is also known as peritendinitis crepitans when the site of the lesion is in the tendons above the upper limit of the tendon sheaths, or tenosynovitis when the synovial lining of the tendon sheath is involved. The lesion is a non-infective inflammatory reaction caused by unaccustomed and arduous exercise of the muscles of the forearm.

Tenosynovitis – A Case Of Mistaken Identity

Diagnosis

Pain, swelling and tenderness may extend up the forearm to the level of the musculo-tendinous junction. Crepitus may be felt over the affected tendons. Some loss of function is usually apparent. The condition does not go on to suppuration. It must be distinguished from other painful afflictions such as golfers' elbow, tennis elbow or arthritis **which are not accepted as prescribed diseases.** It should not be confused with so called writers' cramp which is PD.A4.

Prognosis

The condition usually clears up completely with rest but some cases may become chronic.

Carpal Tunnel Syndrome

Not a prescribed disease in its own right but where it follows an attack of PD.A8 and is considered to be a sequela of such an attack, benefit may be paid in respect of the incapacity/disability arising from the syndrome.

NB *These are the **only** hand and arm conditions for which benefit is payable under the Industrial Injuries Provisions of the Social Security Act 1975.*

The Industrial Injuries Advisory Council (IIAC) has recently announced a new study of upper limb disorders with a view to recommending, if the evidence supports it, some further conditions for addition to the list of prescribed diseases.

The disorders that are to be examined in the new study are tennis elbow (epicondylitis), rotator cuff syndrome, carpal tunnel syndrome, cubital tunnel syndrome and Dupuytren's contracture.

Official Guidance

In attempting to defend claims for upper limb disorders, employers are often caught by the provisions of Guidance Note MS.10 issued in September 1977 by the Health & Safety Executive under the title – **Beat Conditions, Tenosynovitis.**

Prescription And Official Guidance

All are prescribed industrial diseases (although none is a notifiable industrial disease).

Of the beat conditions only beat hand and beat elbow can be described as an upper limb disorder but as they have their own aetiology and have always been largely confined to the mining industry, their connection with tenosynovitis and other similar upper limb disorders is not immediately obvious.

Although failure to conform with the official guidance given by MS.10 is widely pleaded by plaintiffs, it should not be overlooked that this Guidance Note replaced the earlier Chief Employment Medical Adviser's Notes of Guidance issued by the Department of Employment (CEMA) in November 1972 under the same heading – **Beat Conditions/Tenosynovitis.**

Whilst there was occasional reference to occupational cramp and tenosynovitis in the Annual Reports of HM Chief Inspector of Factories, chiefly those in 1965 and 1970, the 1972 Notes of Guidance may be taken as the first official **guidance** on upper limb disorders with the Department of Employment preferring to use the narrow definition **tenosynovitis.**

The 1965 Annual Report suggested that:-

> "Traumatic inflammation of the tendons or tendon sheaths of the hand or muscles inserted in the lower forearm, is a non-infective condition affecting the musculo-tendinous junction or the synovial lining of the tendon sheaths, or the tendons themselves. It is caused by the constant repetition of small quick movements. It may occur in a wide variety of jobs including the packeting of food, typing, operating comptometer and sewing machines, chicken preparing, metal and woodworking, gardening, hop picking, upholstering, net and grommet making. Newcomers to such work and those who resume after a spell away seem specially prone. The clinical features are local pain, swelling, tenderness and sometimes redness. In the absence of complicating factors, the condition usually subsides quickly with rest, but may become chronic after repeated attacks. Alternation of employment is useful in prevention, the workers switching over eg at tea breaks, to work involving different movements. A slowing down of the tempo of work by altering the speed of

Tenosynovitis – A Case Of Mistaken Identity

conveyor belts may have to be considered.

The occupational cramps form a somewhat similar set of conditions which occur in people who have to carry out repeated fine movements such as writers, telegraph operators, cotton twisters, florists, violinists, knitters, seamstresses and the like. The muscles of the hand and forearm are affected resulting in spasm, tremor and pain when carrying out a familiar movement. An underlying psychoneurosis is suspected in many cases but the condition does not often respond to psychological treatment".

The 1970 Annual Report, commenting on the incidence of tenosynovitis in industry, suggested that – "there seems little prospect of reducing the incidence of tenosynovitis in the wide range of jobs which cause it, though some brickworks foremen allow younger men to build up speed on day rates the first week after absence".

In the same report comment was made on tenosynovitis in furniture manufacture, specifically one particular factory. There, arrangements were made for medical supervision of any worker suffering pain in the wrist or arm suggestive of tenosynovitis and, if the diagnosis was confirmed, referral for physiotherapy (heat and rotary massage) for two to three days.

However, nowhere is there any recommendation or guidance to employers.

Chief Employment Medical Adviser's Guidance Note 5 (November 1972) defines tenosynovitis as a non-infectious inflammatory reaction in the tendon sheaths or at the musculo-tendinous junction of the muscles of the forearm. The latter condition (peritendinitis crepitans) is more frequently seen.

The note suggests **tenosynovitis** is an important cause of sick absence. It occurs in many industries but especially those where rapid repetitive twisting and gripping movements are common such as pottery, glaze dipping, brick making, assembly line work and belt conveyor sorting for food canning, press operations and the evisceration and trussing of chickens.

The condition is liable to result from trauma, over-use of the wrist and forearms during repetitive operations, unaccustomed work, alteration in work tempo or from persistent strain. It occurs most often in new employees, on return to work after an absence or on the introduction of a new process or tool which places an unusual strain on muscles.

Guidance Note MS.10 – Issued in September 1977 follows the earlier report almost exactly, suggesting that tenosynovitis is the second commonest prescribed disease in the UK (after dermatitis).

There is however a new section on **Management** but the recommendations are traditional and limited:-

- cessation of causative occupation
- immobilisation
- deep massage.

From the point of view of management and control the document is unhelpful. Its importance lies in the fact that employers involved in a certain number of defined occupations are advised that **tenosynovitis** (and by implication other forms of upper limb disorder) is a risk within some industries. In those circumstances an argument of "lack of knowledge of the problem" is difficult to defend.

1990 Guidance

After much debate and delay the Health & Safety Executive finally published in October 1990 its long awaited replacement for Guidance Note MS.10. Entitled "Work Related Upper Limb Disorders : A Guide to Prevention", the publication provides general advice and guidance for those with duties under the Health & Safety At Work etc. Act 1974 and other relevant legislation.

The publication is the first in a series to be devoted to upper limb disorders and although of general interest to occupational health and safety specialists, workplace health and safety representatives and insurers, the guidance is directed in particular to management and those responsible for production planning.

The term ULD is used deliberately to encompass a range of different conditions affecting the soft tissues of the hand, wrist, arm and shoulder. The use of the term RSI is described as medically imprecise.

Occupational factors which may be causative are described and appropriate preventative measures recommended. In the latter category effective engineering controls and appropriate organisational arrangements are described – these range from ergonomic design of tools, workplaces, equipment and job design to such factors as training, job rotation and work organisation.

Tenosynovitis – A Case Of Mistaken Identity

The Guidance suggests that symptoms in the form of pain, restricted movement of joints and swelling are often gradual although a complex symptom pattern may result. There is evidence of causal link to specific occupation derived from anecdotal reports, workplace surveys, epidemiological studies and ergonomic literature.

Increased risk is associated with:-
- force
- frequency and duration
- awkward posture.

Other contributory factors are:-
- tool design
- compressive stresses
- vibration
- exposure to cold
- poor training.

It is stressed these are all factors that need to be taken into account.

Preventative measures are described and specific risk factors examined. Where risk assessment may be complex it is suggested that expert help should be sought from ergonomic specialists. Ergonomic principles under the headings of work design and organisational arrangements are discussed in detail.

The final section of the Guidance suggests possible solutions. Various factors affect the choice of intervention which must be determined by a systematic investigation of information from a number of sources. No single change is likely to be successful. An ordered control programme is suggested with the object of eliminating or minimising each of the risk factors to achieve the desired solution.

Concentrating on the current state of knowledge, the causes and possible solutions to the specific problems of upper limb disorder, the new Guidance provides the depth and quality of advice that was never apparent from Guidance Note MS.10. As the first definitive guide in a series it raises issues of priority that employers and insurers would be wise not to ignore.

Prescription And Official Guidance

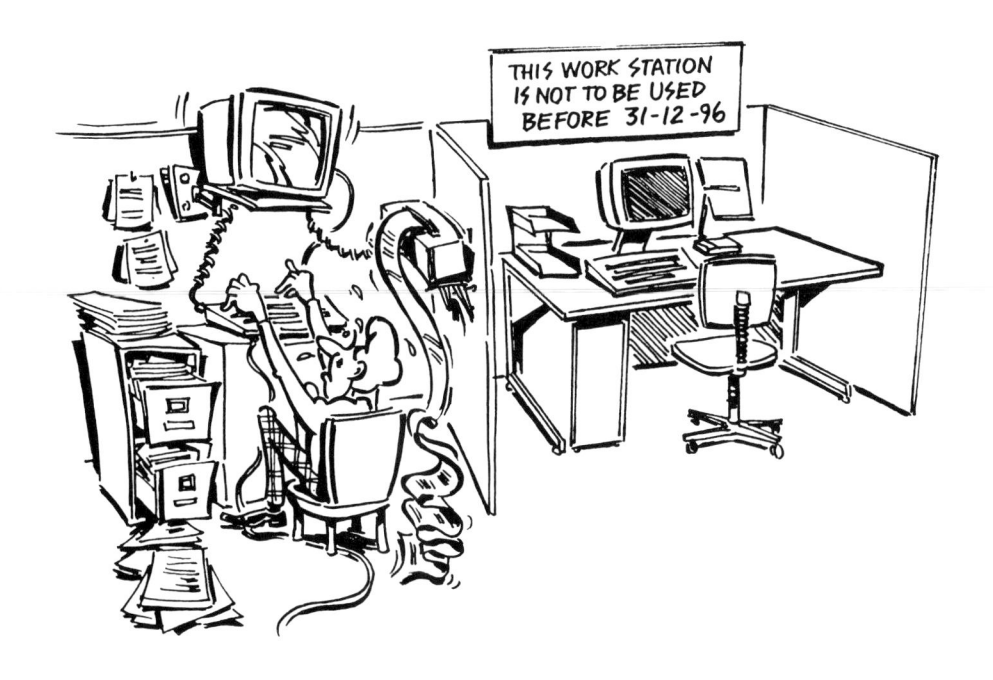

UPPER LIMB DISORDERS – SUMMARY AND CONCLUSIONS

The areas of contention that have been identified may be summarised in broad terms as follows:-

1. Incorrect **definition** – The exact nature of the complaint should be identified and the precise definition used. Emotive terms such as **tenosynovitis** should be avoided unless describing a specific complaint.

2. The potential for **ambiguity** that exists in the **clinical diagnosis** of such disorders. Not all are work related. Medical evidence to establish the **precise** nature of the condition assumes priority – clarity of medical evidence is essential.

3. Genuine disagreement between the disciplines of medicine and ergonomics highlights the need for improved assessment of the physiological and biomechanical effects of **fatigue** in occupations at high risk and the implications of **psychological** or **psychosocial** factors.

4. (a) The high **prevalence** of upper limb disorder in some industries (in particular those mentioned in official publications) despite a substantial reduction in claims for benefit.
   (b) The apparent **correlation** between high rates of upper limb disorder and industries with machine paced jobs or jobs with abnormal wrist positions and forceful movements or grip.
   (c) The adverse effect of **partial automation** resulting in less job variation and possible higher exposure to awkward manual tasks.

5. It is widely accepted that work related upper limb disorder can never be

Upper Limb Disorders – Summary And Conclusions

eradicated entirely but it can be kept to minimal levels. This involves critically appraising the technology used and redesigning work procedures to minimise risk factors.

6. Organisational preventative methods alone (screening, training, job rotation) are insufficient to combat the risk of upper limb disorder. As the causes can be traced primarily to job and equipment design, the organisational features should be used only prior to the introduction of or to complement the work redesign approach.

7. Upper limb disorders are multifactorial in origin, comprising psychosocial and organisational as well as physical components. As a result their prevention requires a broad approach based predominantly on sound ergonomic principles combined with training and appropriate organisational management.

STATUTORY DUTY

Health & Safety at Work etc. Act 1974

This Act is essentially a penal statute. Breach of the rules set out in the Act may invite prosecution but S.47 makes it quite clear that such a breach does not automatically confer a right to a cause of action for damages by the victim except in the case of regulations made under the Act for that specific purpose.

The Factories Act 1961

The Factories Act contains nothing specific. Section 29(1) requires the occupier of factory premises to provide "a safe place of work". Controversy has often arisen as to whether this means the place of work has to be structurally or physically safe, or the work done therein has to be safe. To a great extent this matters not because the requirement is qualified by the words, "so far as reasonably practicable". This is no higher than the common law duty of care.

The Management of Health & Safety At Work Regulations 1992

Whereas the Health & Safety (Display Screen Equipment) Regulations 1992 are specific to one form of process, these Regulations which also came into force on 1 January 1993 are much more general but similar in application.

They have been introduced following the EC Directive entitled Introduction of Measures to Encourage Improvements in the Safety & Health of Workers at Work. They require specific action to be taken to ensure that correct procedures are being undertaken to meet the general requirements of Section 2 of the Health & Safety at Work etc. Act 1974. The Regulations require most employers to undertake the following:-

STATUTORY DUTY

- to assess the health and safety risks to which their employees are exposed (Regulation 3)
- to make effective arrangements for planning, organising, controlling, monitoring and reviewing preventative and protective measures (Regulation 4).

There is also a requirement for health surveillance to be provided where specific health risks are identified in the assessment. (Regulation 5)

Employers must appoint at least one competent person to assist in undertaking the control measures identified in the assessment. (Regulation 6)

The other sections are:-

Regulation 1	Citation, commencement and interpretation.
Regulation 2	Disapplication.
Regulation 7	Serious dangers.
Regulation 8	Information for employees.
Regulation 9	Two or more employers sharing the same workplace.
Regulation 10	Covers the duty of a "host" employer.
Regulation 11	Requires employers to take into account the physical and mental capabilities of employees when entrusting tasks to them.
Regulation 12	Deals with the duty of employees as regards health and safety.
Regulation 13	Covers temporary workers and those on a fixed term contract.
Regulation 14	Exemption certificates.
Regulation 15	Emphasises that a breach of the Regulations does not confer a right of civil action.
Regulation 16	Extension outside of Great Britain.
Regulation 17	Modification.

TENOSYNOVITIS – A CASE OF MISTAKEN IDENTITY

Comments upon the Management of Health and Safety at Work Regulations

These Regulations it seems are designed to add weight to Section 2 of the Health & Safety at Work Act 1974.

In many ways these Regulations encapsulate the common law duty of employers although employers will now be required to **show** that correct procedures are being taken to meet the general requirements of Section 2 of the Health & Safety at Work Act. Apart from identifying areas of health and safety hazards so as to devise ways to combat them, employers are also required to **record** assessment findings and the steps taken to combat hazards.

These Regulations also cover the hazard of upper limb disorders in any area of a workplace.

The Health & Safety (Display Screen Equipment) Regulations 1992 (The Regulations)

(In view of the significance of these Regulations to the subject matter of this book, we deal with them comprehensively).

Background

On 29 May 1990 the European Council of Ministers adopted a Directive laying down minimum health and safety requirements for work with display screen equipment – commonly called visual display units (VDU's) or visual display terminals (VDT's).

The Directive was the fifth individual directive within the meaning of the "framework" directive on "**the introduction of measures to encourage improvements in the safety and health of workers**".

Member states were required to bring into force the necessary **minimum** requirements by 31 December 1992.

Statutory Duty

In the vote on adoption the United Kingdom abstained principally on the grounds that:-

1. the scientific evidence that VDU work is the cause of major health hazards is weak

2. there was insufficient public concern.

To implement the detailed provisions of the European Community Directive, **specific** legislation had to be introduced because the general requirements of the Health & Safety at Work Act are insufficiently detailed to implement the EC Directive.

Together with representatives of the CBI and TUC initial steps taken by the Health & Safety Commission included the formation of a working party with the object of considering what, if any, changes would be required to implement the Directive's provisions.

Following discussion, a consultative document "**Work with Display Screen Equipment – Proposals for Regulations & Guidance**" was issued by the Health & Safety Commission in January 1992. The consultative document contained **draft Regulations** on "the minimum safety and health requirements for work with display screen equipment". It also contained **draft general guidance** to support Regulations. Implementation was proposed by Regulations and Guidance.

Comments from interested parties were invited to reach the Health & Safety Executive by not later than 21 March 1992.

The Regulations were finally laid before Parliament on 16 November 1992 and came into force on 1 January 1993. Copies of the Regulations with Guidance are available from Her Majesty's Stationery Office, price £5.00.

The Regulations are constructed of nine specific sections plus a Schedule setting out minimum requirements for workstations and an explanatory note. The relevant features are:-

> "**1. Citation, commencement, interpretation and application**
> This Regulation, in the main, deals with the **meaning** of certain words or phrases, and **application.** The most significant sections are:-
> (2) In these Regulations:-

Tenosynovitis – A Case Of Mistaken Identity

(a) "display screen equipment" means any alphanumeric or graphic display screen, regardless of the display process involved;
(b) "operator" means a self-employed person who habitually uses display screen equipment as a significant part of his normal work;
(c) "use" means use for or in connection with work;
(d) "user" means an employee who habitually uses display screen equipment as a significant part of his normal work; and
(e) "workstation" means an assembly comprising:-
  (i) display screen equipment (whether provided with software determining the interface between the equipment and its operator or user, a keyboard or any other input device),
  (ii) any optional accessories to the display screen equipment,
  (iii) any disk drive, telephone, modem, printer, document holder, work chair, work desk, work surface or other item peripheral to the display screen equipment, and
  (iv) the immediate work environment around the display screen equipment.
(4) Nothing in these Regulations shall apply to or in relation to:-
  (a) drivers' cabs or control cabs for vehicles or machinery;
  (b) display screen equipment on board a means of transport;
  (c) display screen equipment mainly intended for public operation;
  (d) portable systems not in prolonged use;
  (e) calculators, cash registers or any equipment having a small data or measurement display required for direct use of the equipment; or
  (f) "window typewriters".

Regulation 2 requires employers to perform an **analysis** of workstations to evaluate health hazards:-

2. **Analysis of workstations to assess and reduce risks**
   "(1) Every employer shall perform a suitable and sufficient analysis of those workstations which -
     (a) (regardless of who has provided them) are used for the purposes of his undertaking by users; or
     (b) have been provided by him and are used for the purposes of his undertaking by operators,

STATUTORY DUTY

for the purpose of assessing the health and safety risks to which those persons are exposed in consequence of that use.

(2) Any assessment made by an employer in pursuance of paragraph (1) shall be reviewed by him if -

(a) there is reason to suspect that it is no longer valid; or

(b) there has been a significant change in the matters to which it relates;

and where as a result of any such review changes to an assessment are required, the employer concerned shall make them.

(3) The employer shall reduce the risks identified in consequence of an assessment to the lowest extent reasonably practicable.

(4) The reference in paragraph (3) to "an assessment" is a reference to an assessment made by the employer concerned in pursuance of paragraph (1) and changed by him where necessary in pursuance of paragraph (2)".

Regulation 3 sets time limits for **action**:-

3. Requirements for workstations

"(1) Every employer shall ensure that any workstation first put into service on or after 1st January 1993 which -

(a) (regardless of who has provided it) may be used for the purposes of his undertaking by users; or

(b) has been provided by him and may be used for the purposes of his undertaking by operators,

meets the requirements laid down in the Schedule to these Regulations to the extent specified in paragraph 1 thereof.

(2) Every employer shall ensure that any workstation first put into service on or before 31st December 1992 which -

(a) (regardless of who provided it) may be used for the purposes of his undertaking by users; or

(b) was provided by him and may be used for the purposes of his undertaking by operators,

meets the requirements laid down in the Schedule to these Regulations to the extent specified in paragraph 1 thereof not later than 31st December 1996."

Tenosynovitis – A Case Of Mistaken Identity

4. **Daily work routine of users**

    "Every employer shall so plan the activities of users at work in his undertaking that their daily work on display screen equipment is periodically interrupted by such breaks or changes of activity as reduce their workload at that equipment."

    Guidance Note 45 (c) and (d) advocates short frequent breaks say 5-10 minutes after 50-60 minutes of continuous screen and/or keyboard work, if possible away from the screen.

5. **Eyes and eyesight**

    The requirements here are arguably the most controversial but they have little bearing upon this publication.

    Regulations 6 and 7 require the employer to provide **training** and **information** on health and safety to a user of a workstation and to tell him/her what steps have been or are being taken to comply with the Regulations.

6. **Provision of training**

    "(1) Where a person -
    - (a) is already a user on the date of coming into force of these Regulations; or
    - (b) is an employee who does not habitually use display screen equipment as a significant part of his normal work but is to become a user in the undertaking in which he is already employed,

    his employer shall ensure that he is provided with adequate health and safety training in the use of any workstation upon which he may be required to work.

    (2) Every employer shall ensure that each user at work in his undertaking is provided with adequate health and safety training whenever the organisation of any workstation in that undertaking upon which he may be required to work is substantially modified."

7. **Provision of information**

    "(1) Every employer shall ensure that operators and users at work in his undertaking are provided with adequate information about -
    - (a) all aspects of health and safety relating to their workstations; and
    - (b) such measures taken by him in compliance with his duties under

Statutory Duty

Regulations 2 and 3 as relate to them and their work.

(2) Every employer shall ensure that users at work in his undertaking are provided with adequate information about such measures taken by him in compliance with his duties under Regulations 4 and 6(2) as relate to them and their work.

(3) Every employer shall ensure that users employed by him are provided with adequate information about such measures taken by him in compliance with his duties under Regulations 5 and 6(1) as relate to them and their work."

Regulations 8 and 9 cover **Exemption certificates** (8) and **Extensions outside Great Britain** (9).

Comments upon the Display Screen Regulations

The Regulations closely follow the provisions of the Directive. Scope has been allowed for future technological advances. Interpretation is provided by the detailed Guidance.

The Regulations impose upon employers major new statutory responsibilities although the Health & Safety Commission believes that the principal risks associated with display screen equipment – physical (musculo-skeletal) problems, visual fatigue and mental stress – can largely be overcome by the application of **established** ergonomic principles. Such risks apply to many tasks apart from screen work.

The implications of the Directive are nevertheless far reaching and will undoubtedly necessitate a major change in workplace practice although may not involve the major cost at first envisaged.

The main areas of contention revealed by the specific and general observations of interested parties may be summarised as follows:-

1. the Regulations do not require **all** display screen equipment workstations to meet the minimum requirements

2. full eye tests are not available to **all** display screen equipment workers

3. the definition of a display screen equipment worker is too restrictive

4. the guidance on screen breaks is too shallow.

Tenosynovitis – A Case Of Mistaken Identity

These criticisms arise largely from those organisations representing the employees' point of view suggesting that the Regulations implement neither the spirit nor the letter of the Directive. Against that the employers' representatives express serious concern about the **absolute** nature of many of the new duties. Several of the submissions made by both employer and union criticise the comprehensiveness of the Regulations and the lack of consistency which exists between them and other existing and proposed requirements.

The implications for the **insurance industry** are obvious as a breach of the Regulations will give rise to a civil cause of action. It is of concern to both employers and insurers that full compliance with the new Regulations is not without difficulty. A further dilemma for employers who already have workstations in place arises from the problems of whether to take advantage of the 4 year period of compliance allowed by the Regulations, using the new Regulations as a defence to any action for personal injury brought by an employee within that period, or whether to be guided by the effect of the judgement in McSherry -v- British Telecom which criticised the employer's system on posture and seating. The conflict is clear.

It is important however that the requirement to **assess** display screen workstations and **evaluate** the risk to safety and health should not be confused with the requirement to ensure that workstations meet **specified minimum requirements.** The **minimum requirements** do not apply to workstations, in service before 1993, until 31 December 1996 but the requirement to **assess the risks** is applicable to **all** workstations, now that the Regulations have been implemented.

Screen display work is a complex area but remains high profile. Employers who fail to implement the new Regulations face the risk of penalties in a number of forms including increased insurance premiums.

INVESTIGATION AND CLAIMS HANDLING

Investigation

No matter how diligent an employer may be in terms of risk assessment and management it is likely that claims will still arise that will require investigation and such investigations require careful consideration.

Following receipt of a Letter of Claim it is the normal practice of insurers and/or their solicitors fully to investigate all the known facts at the earliest opportunity and to take steps to obtain appropriate medical evidence.

Investigations focus on two main areas:-

1. **Causation** – Was the employment causative of the injury?

2. **Liability** – Is the employer legally liable for the damage sustained?

Causation is determined by medical evidence – liability by thorough investigation and careful consideration of the evidence.

These issues are examined in detail.

Causation & Medical Evidence

Although the claimant's representatives (usually an experienced firm of solicitors) may be prepared at the outset to release a copy of their medical evidence, it is the normal procedure for the defendant employers to obtain their own report. In practice this is done by the insurers who will normally use a reliable independent orthopaedic surgeon of their own choosing. Permission for a medical examination to take place must firstly be obtained from the claimant and/or the claimant's representative. Full instructions to the chosen medical specialist **must** include written permission for access to the general

Tenosynovitis – A Case Of Mistaken Identity

practitioner and hospital notes (where applicable) and to the works medical records.

Most experienced consultants who have prepared reports for defendants on a regular basis dealing with the causation of upper limb disorder complaints are aware of what information is required by defendants. The report should include and comment upon all the following points:-

- personal details of the claimant including social activities
- details of claimant's medical history
- full details of the claimant's working history
- a full history of symptoms from the date of first occurrence, when and to whom reported, action taken and details of treatment given
- details of present complaints and their effect on work and leisure activities
- a full clinical examination with referral for x-ray examination where considered necessary
- consideration of hospital, GP and works medical records
- an opinion as to the nature and cause of the disease and the period in which it may have occurred
- an assessment of present disability and capability for work
- the effect on working capacity and the prospects of alternative employment
- prognosis – ie whether deterioration or resolution may be expected.

In order to produce a comprehensive medical report, the chosen medical specialist must fully understand the system of work and consider whether the action taken by the employer, both before and after the event, was reasonable. Ideally he should visit the workplace to see the system of work for himself – alternatively have a full report describing the system in detail together with photographs.

A supplementary report might consider:-

- whether the system of reporting complaints was reasonable
- whether action taken by the medical centre was adequate
- whether it was foreseeable that complaints might arise from the particular process and whether any form of warning ought to have

INVESTIGATION AND CLAIMS HANDLING

   been given – if so what form should the warning have taken
- whether any delay in reporting may have aggravated the complaint
- whether there was any pre-disposition to this type of complaint (this may have some relevance to future wage loss).

Where causation becomes a relevant argument the role of the medical witness is important. Sometimes the potential cost of a claim justifies two medical specialists being instructed.

Liability

A comprehensive investigation into liability should establish the following information:-

- the age and normal occupation of the claimant (where not already known)
- the date of commencement of employment
- the date and time the complaint was first reported
- to whom reported
- the exact nature of the report
- the action, if any, which was taken
- a full description of the process upon which the claimant was employed when the complaint first arose
- the length of time the claimant had been employed in that process
- the normal length of the working day and the number and nature of breaks allowed
- whether rotation was an option – either between members of a team or squad working essentially on the same process, or rotation with workers on a different process
- the nature of any **other** process upon which the claimant may on occasion have been temporarily employed
- the length of time spent in any alternative process
- the extent of **repetitive and forceful movement** in **any process** on which the claimant was employed
- whether difficulties had been experienced by the claimant over a

Tenosynovitis – A Case Of Mistaken Identity

    period of time and if so, the dates involved
- whether such difficulties had been reported, to whom complaints were made and whether such complaints were acted upon
- whether there had been complaints from any other workers employed in the process (other than the usual general grumbles which are a normal part of the working scene) – ie whether there was a history of complaint
- whether a reasonable change of process could have been adopted to alleviate any difficulties complained of
- whether a formal policy of transfer exists on receipt of a report or complaint
- formal details of absences and whether supported by a doctor's sick note
- whether the condition may have been caused or contributed to by faulty tools or equipment
- if so, how long such faults had existed, whether faults had been reported and to whom such faults were reported
- whether other claims have arisen from the same process – ie is there a history of claims
- whether there exists any formal system of education, instruction, training and warning (both pre-employment and early symptom reporting)
- whether there exists a regular system of medical examinations
- whether there has been any correspondence/recommendations from the Health and Safety Inspectors regarding precautionary measures to be taken
- details of sports/hobbies that may have been undertaken by the claimant
- anecdotal evidence of cause.

If necessary the opportunity should be taken to examine relevant documents such as works notices, employee hand books or hand-outs and minutes of safety committee meetings where available.

Investigation And Claims Handling

Claims Handling

There are a number of fundamental issues which must be determined.

The policy cover, particularly periods of relevant insurance, must be checked. There may be other employers and/or insurers than the current insurer who should be contributing towards any proposed payment of damages. However upper limb disorders are not normally insidious in nature and can usually be attributed to a particular period in time.

The employment history should be checked. The complaint may pre-date commencement of employment. Current employment may only have aggravated rather than caused the condition.

Given that hand and arm complaints take many different forms – not all of which are occupational in origin – it is important to establish at the outset that the process on which the claimant was employed was **causative** of the injury sustained.

The exact form and nature of the injury sustained, its origins, progress and prognosis, all of which are necessary to determine not only **causation** but **damages** can usually only be established by medical evidence.

It is likely that the claimant's medical evidence will suggest that the process, or at least one of the processes on which the claimant was employed, was the offending process as otherwise it is unlikely that the report will have been disclosed. Refusal by the claimant's representative to disclose a medical report or an indication that the report is not to be relied upon is usually evidence of the fact that the report is unfavourable.

In practice the claimant could obtain several reports (without the knowledge of the employers or the insurers) and then choose to rely upon the report which is the most favourable to the case.

This must be contrasted with the position of the defendant employer. The claimant and his/her representative are fully aware that the defendant employer/insurer has obtained a report and from whom (permission for access to the medical notes being required). If thereafter they fail or refuse to disclose the report at the claimant's request, the claimant will be aware that the report is almost certainly unfavourable to the defendants and may seek to impose restrictions on the obtaining of further medical evidence.

Alternatively there may be merit in the defendants disclosing at an early stage a **favourable** medical report more especially where an argument on

Tenosynovitis – A Case Of Mistaken Identity

causation may support doubtful liability. There are no hard and fast rules. Outside of litigation the question of disclosure of medical evidence and at what stage is one of judgement and discretion dependent upon the facts of the individual case.

If having exhausted medical enquiries, causation is established the next element to be considered is that of **liability**.

The defendants' evidence may show that:-

1. they did not know and could not reasonably have foreseen that an employee was exposed to risk

2. their system of working was safe, was arranged and conducted in accordance with minimum standards to be expected in the industry and was properly enforced.

In support the defendants may rely upon the absence of any or any significant injury or complaint relating specifically to the condition complained of.

These facts can only be determined by detailed enquiry in association with a perusal of all relevant employment and medical records.

Plainly, if as a result of enquiry, there is clear evidence of previous similar injury or complaint arising from the process to which the enquiry is directed, the employer will be deemed to have **knowledge** of the potential problems for individuals arising from the process.

If the defendant employer is part of a large group, knowledge of a potentially unsafe process within that **group** may be a factor.

Should a further claim arise thereafter from the same offending process, the defendant employer, in order to defeat a common law action, must be in a position to show that he took some positive step – broadly either that he took action to alter or amend the process or if that was not practicable, that the employee was informed of the risk.

If the employer, having knowledge of a possible risk, did **nothing,** it is likely that he will be found liable.

The action to be taken by an employer to alleviate a risk must be considered on the merits of the individual case balanced against such matters as the extent, potential and nature of the injury arising, the cost of effective alterations to the process and the necessary effect that such changes may have on production. The employer should not be liable if the cost of change involved an

INVESTIGATION AND CLAIMS HANDLING

unreasonable additional financial burden.

When considering whether action could have been taken by the employer or what action was taken to reduce the hazard, it is often helpful to obtain the evidence of an independent consulting engineer. Indeed it may be essential where the claimant has obtained his own engineer's report – if only to deal with any comments that may be made by the claimant's expert. Permission for an on-site inspection should only be granted after the claimant has set out, with sufficient particularity, all his complaints. As with the medical specialist, the chosen expert should be experienced in handling claims for work related upper limb disorder.

Preferably photographs showing the system or process should accompany the report and where possible **the expert should try the process for himself** to determine whether any degree of force or effort is involved.

Many engineers now have access to video equipment and can produce a short video film of the relevant operation which is admissible in evidence in any court action. A video film must however be used carefully. Whilst it can illustrate technique and repetition it cannot always demonstrate the degree of force and effort required.

If, after having considered all the relevant technical evidence, the conclusion is that it was **not** feasible for the employer to have altered his process to any material degree or that whatever steps **were taken** were in all the circumstances adequate, the question of **informing** or **warning** the employee becomes relevant.

Engineering evidence may conclude that the process, although producing evidence of upper limb disorder, was inherently safe or was a practice followed throughout the industry generally.

The nature of warnings has already been discussed; the effect of warnings must now be considered.

Clearly if the employer has knowledge, and he is unable to amend the process, a warning is the appropriate next step. All that means is that the employee should have been informed to report for medical attention at the first sign of distress.

Failure to warn does not however necessarily mean that there is liability.

The dates of onset and first reporting of symptoms must be checked. If the dates coincide then effectively the employee has taken precisely the action that he would have been told to take thus nullifying the effect of warning. If the

TENOSYNOVITIS – A CASE OF MISTAKEN IDENTITY

employer followed the generally accepted practice and referred the employee for more specialised treatment his duty is discharged. If there was a delay between the onset of symptoms and the date on which the claimant first reported then the employer is open to an allegation of aggravation of the symptoms by allowing the claimant to continue working (see Burgess -v- Thorn page 125).

The next step is to investigate the position following the claimant's resumption of work.

Medical discharge (a Final Certificate from the General Practitioner) allowing resumption of normal duties should be available, alternatively, a doctor's note suggesting resumption of light duties pending full recovery. The actual position must be checked against the personnel files to determine whether recommendations of this nature have been followed. If they have not, and the employee has been returned to his pre-injury duties too early causing additional absence, the employer could well be liable for a recurrence of the initial injury.

Where the employer **did not** have knowledge of previous injury or complaint the burden on the employer is lighter. The question then is whether he should have **foreseen** that the process on which the claimant was employed was likely to give rise to the **kind of injury** sustained. If foreseeability is **established** the employer is placed in the same position as if he had actual "knowledge" and it must be shown that in the absence of any positive step to lessen the risk to the employee, some other remedial action such as education or warning was taken.

If there is doubt the advice and guidance of an expert engineer on the question of **foreseeability** should be obtained.

In the absence of either knowledge or foreseeability there is no **specific** obligation upon the employer to take **additional** precautions to prevent the onset of upper limb complaints **over and above** the normal requirements of health & safety legislation such as the safety requirements of Section 14 of the Factories Act. Nevertheless the employer who has in place a Health & Safety Policy which anticipates such contingencies arising and has already taken steps to implement a system of education, warning and early reporting of symptoms is more likely to have met his duty of care to his employees.

Finally, consideration must be given to potential lay witnesses either currently employed or retired who can give evidence on some or all of the issues, particularly historical details. They will need to be interviewed and statements taken.

INVESTIGATION AND CLAIMS HANDLING

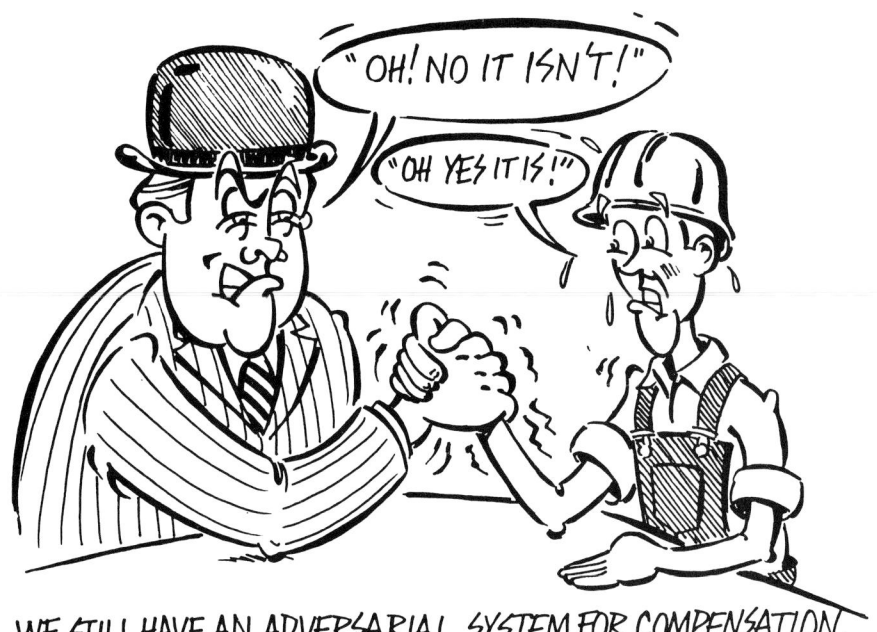

WE STILL HAVE AN ADVERSARIAL SYSTEM FOR COMPENSATION.

Summary of Evidence

A relatively simple method of reviewing the evidence in claims for upper limb disorder is to summarise the relevant facts in the form of a schedule or table. An example of the kind of schedule envisaged follows but may be varied to suit individual requirements. Such a schedule should include all relevant information – dates, event or complaint, action taken – and a comparison made with existing case law.

It should not be forgotten that claims may be decided on the evidence of witnesses rather than on medical and/or ergonomic literature however learned, deep or carefully prepared. The role of good witness material therefore remains of critical importance and this includes the careful and meticulous recording of evidence in a written form.

As we still have an adversarial system for compensation of injuries, there are bound to be conflicts between employers and employees on causation, liability and extent of damages. However, most employers adopt a reasonable attitude of: "investigate, if we have not met our duty of care compensation should be paid". There is rarely a desire to contest liability without good cause.

Tenosynovitis – A Case Of Mistaken Identity

Example of Summary

Claimant: _____

Age: _____

Occupation: _____

Date of Birth: _____

Date	Event	Action
07/06/76	Commenced employment - Box Room Dept (Leeds Factory) various jobs – feeding, stripping, taking off.	Any training (check)
June 1986	First noticed aching left wrist (feeding)	Allegedly reported to works nurse

NB   ? when – no report

Date	Event	Action
June 1989	Pains left wrist at night with discomfort	Consulted own doctor - referred to hospital
14/07/89	Reported to Works Surgery – complained of swelling – left wrist – burning, tingling, numbness	Strap provided - returned to work same job – Advised to see GP

NB   *No further visits to Works Surgery.*

Date	Event	Action
November 1989	Hospital treatment - carpal tunnel syndrome diagnosed	Splint & electric treatment
February 1990	Follow up hospital treatment	No improvement
16/04/90	Ceased work (operation)	Doctors note decompression of carpal (symptoms improved)
26/06/90	Returned to work (Hospital discharge)	Where employed (check)

NB   *No education or warnings to workforce – leather wrist straps introduced September 1989 – no work rotation.*

INVESTIGATION AND CLAIMS HANDLING

18/09/90	Letter of Claim Alleged RSI Alleged negligence	Referred to insurers
26/09/90	Letter of Claim acknowledged (no further response)	
05/11/90	Investigation report - conclude not foreseeable	Deny liability (obtain medical evidence first)
05/03/91	Defendants medical report	Reasonable recovery following operation - constitutional – not work related.

NB *Liability denied – possible proceedings.*

Litigation And Case Law

It is appropriate that we leave litigation and case law until last in our considerations. We are more concerned with prevention. However, there will be occasions where genuine disputes arise and have to be resolved; litigation cannot always be avoided. Once litigation is commenced, both plaintiff and defendant will wish to present the best case possible.

The outcome of litigation is often determined by case law, a term which needs to be closely defined. The decisions of the House of Lords are binding on all courts. The decisions of the Court of Appeal are binding on lower courts (courts of first instance). The decision of a lower court is not binding on another lower court although it may be of persuasive value. It is important to bear in mind that the court can only reach a decision on the facts presented to it. Thus a poorly presented case will undoubtedly produce a result adverse to the party who has not done his homework.

We consider under this heading four essential elements:-

1. The conduct of the reasonable and prudent employer.

2. A review of case law.

3. The identifiable legal issues.

4. Damages – examples of court and other awards.

1. The Conduct Of The Reasonable And Prudent Employer

Generally speaking, an employer owes a duty of care to provide a safe place of work for his employees whilst acting in the course of their employment with him.

Litigation And Case Law

The standard of such duty of care required in law, and which is of particular relevance to claims for industrial disease, was defined by Mr Justice Swanwick in the case of STOKES -v- GUEST, KEEN & NETTLEFORD (BOLTS & NUTS) LTD – (1968 1 WLR)

> "The overall test is still the conduct of the reasonable and prudent employer, taking positive thought for the safety of his workers in the light of what he knows or ought to know; where there is a recognised and general practice which has been followed for a substantial period in similar circumstances without mishap, he is entitled to follow it, unless in the light of common sense or newer knowledge it is clearly bad; but, where there is developing knowledge, he must keep reasonably abreast of it and not be too slow to apply it; and where he has in fact greater than average knowledge of the risks, he may be thereby obliged to take more than the average or standard precautions. He must weigh up the risk in terms of the likelihood of injury occurring and the potential consequences if it does; and he must balance against this the probable effectiveness of the precautions that can be taken to meet it and the expense and inconvenience they involve. If he is found to have fallen below the standard to be properly expected of a reasonable and prudent employer in these respects, he is negligent."

2. A Review Of Case Law

In reviewing existing case law the broad comments of Mr Justice Swanwick, whilst they express important principles (of equal application in any case of industrial disease) serve only as the basis for further consideration of upper limb disorder claims.

Additionally a number of other court decisions have been identified as having some bearing on the general conduct and outcome of litigated claims for upper limb disorder.

The main points arising from these cases are stressed and are largely the specific comments of the court itself.

Tenosynovitis – A Case Of Mistaken Identity

WITHERS -v- PERRY CHAIN
COURT OF APPEAL
JULY 1961

In this dermatitis case the Court of Appeal held that the employers were under no duty to dismiss or to refuse to employ an adult employee who wished to do a job merely because there might be some slight risk to the employee in doing the work.

If the employer were to conceal the risk or fail to give the employee information which he had and which might help her to evaluate it properly, there might perhaps be a liability or there might be a case where the employer impliedly warranted that the job was safe for the employee.

KOSSINSKI -v- CHRYSLER (UK) LTD
COURT OF APPEAL
12 NOVEMBER 1973

"I am completely unsatisfied that they were failing in their duty of reasonable care in the only aspect relied on – The works surgery should have investigated what work the plaintiff could do without harming himself and arranged the matter accordingly .... such a submission imposes upon the employers in the circumstances of this case a duty going far beyond the duty of reasonable care."

"It requires no authority to illustrate the cogency of the proposition that the duty of reasonable care does not impose upon an employer the necessity of saying to an employee :

'You are not fit for this properly-planned and entirely safe work because of your own physical condition, and therefore, despite your own desire to continue at it, we must dismiss you.' "

"In certain cases a duty of warning by the employers may arise, but it must depend upon the circumstances of the case."

Litigation And Case Law

"I do not think that these defendant employers were failing in their duty when they allowed this man to continue at the work he was doing."

"When the man himself made no complaint, I do not think it was incumbent on the employers to conduct an investigation as to what, if any, other alternative work was available for him or to give him such warning that if he wanted to continue with his work he would do so at his peril."

NELSON -v- PLESSEY
CANTLEY J – NEWCASTLE
15 MARCH 1977

"I do not consider they can be criticised for taking her back to resume work."

"......... would have been a good idea to say 'Try your work but if you have any trouble let us know at once.' That seems to me to be a very practical sensible suggestion."

PRESLAND -v- G W PADLEY LTD
TUDOR EVANS J – LINCOLN
29 JANUARY 1979

"...an employer is under a duty in cases where the nature of the work carries an inherent, specific and not insignificant risk of a servant developing an industrial disease or condition to tell the servant at the beginning of the employment about the risk in order to allow the servant the option whether to embark on the employment or not."

Tenosynovitis – A Case Of Mistaken Identity

"On the facts, the issues are whether a warning was necessary, if it was given whether it was adequate. Finally if no adequate warning was given whether the failure was a cause of the plaintiff's damage."

"The essential question is whether the warning she received from Mr Walker was sufficient to bring home to her that aches and pains in the hands were sufficiently serious to require treatment and could lead to a disabling condition."

"... plaintiff is entitled to succeed and on the grounds that the defendants failed to give her a specific warning of the risks of the onset of tenosynovitis and because the warning which was given did not sufficiently bring home to her the need to visit the nurse in the event of trouble in her hands and wrists."

WHITE -v- HOLBROOK PRECISION CASTINGS
COURT OF APPEAL
10 APRIL 1984

In this vibration white finger claim, the Court of Appeal in upholding the decision of the judge at first instance came to the following conclusion:-

"What should an employer tell a prospective employee about the risks he will expose himself to if he takes the job? Generally speaking, if a job has risks to health and safety which are not common knowledge but of which an employer knows, or ought to know and against which he cannot guard by taking precautions, then he should tell anyone to whom he is offering the job what those risks are if, on the information then available to him, knowledge of those risks would be likely to affect the decision of a sensible, level-headed prospective employee about accepting the offer."

Litigation And Case Law

BURGESS -v- THORN – BRISTOW J
ROYAL COURTS OF JUSTICE
11 MAY 1983

"....it would have been simple to warn the Insertion Line workers that if they started having pain in the wrist or arm, they must report it at once and consult their doctor, because it might well indicate the presence of a condition which if dealt with promptly would be innocuous, but if not dealt with might soon become serious enough to require surgery."

(Defendants) " were in breach of their duty to take reasonable care for her safety in failing to give her the warning which would probably have meant that her tenosynovitis would not have required the decompression operation, with its unhappy result...".

TREE -v- M K ELECTRICS – TAYLOR J
ROYAL COURTS OF JUSTICE
9 NOVEMBER 1984

"The medical evidence is that if the relevant part is rested at an early stage the probability is that recovery will take place. Where the trouble is caused by repetitive movements, if those are stopped when the early symptoms are evident then again the probability is that the disease will not develop and will not become chronic."

"One is left with this situation, that these are jobs which are highly repetitive and which do as a matter of general knowledge in the industry carry some risk to some people of the contraction of tenosynovitis."

"It is for the employer who can take the longer view and whose duty it is to study, not only what is happening on his own shop floor but what is happening in the other factories of the same company and what has been known to happen in other places of similar industries, to lay out the work; lay out a system of work and take reasonable care for his employees in accordance with that knowledge."

"... the defendants were failing to give the kind of warning and the kind of reasonable care for their employees which they ought to have given, in a general way as to their general system."

**LANE -v- SUN VALLEY POULTRY – BUSH J
BIRMINGHAM
28 MARCH 1985**

"Now the fact that you cannot tell beforehand those likely to suffer from the condition, and the fact that those likely to be affected is a very small percentage of the workforce does not mean that the work should not be carried out at all."

"The precaution that a good employer should take is to warn his workforce that if they should experience any pain or discomfort in the wrist, then they should go to the Work's Surgery and/or see their own General Practitioner, and a good employer should see that if pain of this kind is complained of, then the worker not only has medical treatment but if still able to work is put on different work."

"I am satisfied that even had a warning been given in suitable terms the plaintiff would have taken the employment."

"... what happened, namely that she reported to the Surgery and stopped work when she had a pain in her wrist, was what would have happened if she had the warning contended for from the beginning."

"In my view the warning given to the plaintiff by the defendants was adequate in the sense that it brought to her mind – and it was given, I am satisfied, in the induction period – the difficulties that might arise as a result of this work and also brought clearly to her mind the fact that if she had a pain in her wrist or thumb, she should go to the Surgery and stop work, and in fact that is what happened.

In the circumstances there was no further step the employers could take, in my view to protect the plaintiff."

"... a person is either going to get tenosynovitis or not. The cutting down period of work does not make any difference."

"In the end I was still left with the problem that only a very few get tenosynovitis and you cannot predict beforehand which ones."

**PEPALL & OTHERS -v- THORN CONSUMER ELECTRONICS – WOOLF J
ROYAL COURTS OF JUSTICE
20 DECEMBER 1985**

"Where the defendants did fall down on the duty which they owed to their employees to exercise reasonable care for their safety, in general, was because the steps which ought to have been taken to combat the risk of tenosynovitis required a relatively sophisticated programme of educating and warning employees, which at the relevant time Mr Shaw had neither the experience nor the knowledge to devise. The problem needed consideration and implementation by management at a high level and on the evidence which is before me this did not occur."

"From a practical point of view, it would be unreasonable to expect the defendants to give their employees a warning before they start work at the defendants' Gosport factory. When employees are taken into employment, it is not known precisely upon what job they will be engaged..."

Tenosynovitis – A Case Of Mistaken Identity

> "The employer's duty can be satisfactorily discharged initially if he gives a proper warning before the work having the inherent risk is begun."

> "In adopting the general approach indicated by Bristow J (see Burgess), I would emphasise it is particularly important that the warning should contain an explanation of why it is necessary to report."

> "What was needed was, not only one warning, coupled with an explanation, but a regular education process, bringing home to the employee the particular steps which could be taken by the employee having regard to the nature of his or her work to reduce the risks."

> "... the individual plaintiffs are only entitled to succeed if they can establish, either that this breach of duty was causative of the injuries which they allege they suffered, or there was some other breach of duty which was responsible."

NB *The judge found that whilst there was no duty upon this particular employer to warn* **prospective** *employees of the risk of tenosynovitis (or related conditions), because at that stage, which was prior to training, it would not be known what work a given employee would be doing, nevertheless he considered that there was a duty upon the employer to warn and* **to continue to warn** *when a person was put on work that involved an* **"inherent, specific and not insignificant risk"** *of developing tenosynovitis or a similar condition.*

It will be noted that there will be occasions when the employee should be removed from the process, even if this involves dismissal (but see Withers -v- Perry Chain, page 122).

LITIGATION AND CASE LAW

WYETH -v- THAMES CASE
COURT OF APPEAL
3 JUNE 1986

Quoting judge at first instance, Mr Patrick Bennett QC:-

"It is common ground between the parties that warning the workforce of the dangers of repetitive work, making sure that there was a sufficient rotation of the work to give the girls a spell from the more taxing tasks and making sure that the girls did not work at so rapid a pace that they made the likelihood of injury greater were factors which the defendants had to consider in the discharge of their duty."

The Court of Appeal concluded that:-

"...the plaintiff was warned, as the other girls were warned, that the situation continued to prevail in which the defendants perfectly reasonably believed that they had done all they possibly could to encourage the workforce to accede to the specifications of the job, in the interests of their own safety as well as in the interests of getting the work performed."

WHITNALL -v- CULROSE FOODS – JUDGE J
ROYAL COURTS OF JUSTICE
13 JUNE 1990

"Tenosynovitis and the sort of working conditions in which it might be caused should have been known by employers such as these defendants by **1982 if not earlier.**"

"These employers could not possibly have known whether any of the staff actually employed in new dispatch, and if so which of them, might have been **susceptible** to tenosynovitis."

Tenosynovitis – A Case Of Mistaken Identity

"In my judgment the employers' duty to take reasonable care of their staff was not performed by doing nothing at all. There should have been a degree of alertness to complaints and education of staff and supervisors about the possible risks. In this context education does not involve lengthy lectures; nothing of the sort – just sensible information, advice, to this effect : if your wrists play you up or your fingers are painful, go and see whoever it might be, supervisor, safety officer or trade union representative and tell them."

"Such a system would not, of course, have avoided the **onset** of symptoms in a **susceptible** employee. It would have enabled the **susceptible** employee to **report** the onset of symptoms."

"The defendants' system for protecting employees who might be susceptible to tenosynovitis was inadequate."

".... even if the defendants had employed a proper system for education, advice and information it would have made no difference to the plaintiff who would have refused to tell the defendants about her condition and would have ignored advice ...."

"In practical terms, even if the defendants had no system of the kind required for this particular job .... the offer of different employment at various times after March 1983 would have amounted to sufficient compliance with any obligation owed to the plaintiff, if and when the defendants had become alert to her particular susceptibilities."

LITIGATION AND CASE LAW

GLEESON-BARTLETT -v- E B PACKERS – JUPP J
ROYAL COURTS OF JUSTICE
31 JULY 1990

1. Plaintiff suffered a transient attack of tenosynovitis with swelling of the wrist.

2. Plaintiff not suitable for the job and had to be told so in stages by proper warning.

3. She received proper medical advice.

4. The system of work was carefully planned and efficiently implemented.

5. Such system had stood the test of time without undue risk.

6. There was a system of warning new starters.

7. The training was more than adequate.

8. Insignificant risk of tenosynovitis – no great force required and not highly repetitive.

9. Management took all reasonable precautions to prevent such risk.

10. Plaintiff's actions in breach of instruction not to work beyond point of aching wrist or forearm and to report when they felt trouble.

LAWLER – v – IMI YORKSHIRE COPPER TUBE LTD
JUDGE LACHS
LIVERPOOL COUNTY COURT
1990

Although this was a deafness judgement handed down in the County Court it is worth noting the comments of the judge on the employer's efforts at hearing conservation to avoid hearing damage:-

"This calls for strong, persuasive, imaginative, sustained propaganda. More than a short talk and shorter films; more than a notice in a pay packet; more even than a notice stuck up in a Clocking on Office."

(but see WHITNALL -v- CULROSE FOODS, pages 129-130)

FOX -v- CHAMPION SPARKING PLUG CO LTD
LIVERPOOL COUNTY COURT
7 NOVEMBER 1990

"Section 29 can apply." (Reference to Factories Act)

"I do not accept the argument that because a place of work causes a person to suffer an injury it necessarily follows that the place of work is unsafe."

"Plaintiff must show a material serious risk of injury before it can be said her place of work was unsafe." (In agreement with Counsel).

"I do not think I am justified in concluding that any injury she may have suffered represented a repetitive strain syndrome."

"I do not accept that there is ample evidence ....."(to conclude that there was a significant risk of which the defendants should have made themselves aware).

"If risk significant, it is not necessary for there to have been a previous incident. If this unsafe system renders place of work unsafe lack of incident not a bar to plaintiff's success."

"Plaintiff is not entitled to say there is a degree of risk in such a process in absence of history of injury."

"... not satisfied that the plaintiff has proved that at her place of work there was a reasonably foreseeable cause of injury...."

Litigation And Case Law

"... not been proved that the plaintiff's place of work was unsafe and therefore the issue as to whether or not the defendants took such steps as were reasonably practicable to make it safe does not arise."

"The allegations of common law negligence fail."

PING & OTHERS -v- ESSELTE LETRASET LTD
ASHFORD COUNTY COURT
8 JULY 1991

"In my judgment the defendants ought reasonably to have been aware that the **inspection and packaging** activities of the type upon which the plaintiffs were engaged could give rise to the sort of injuries which they allege they suffered."

"I therefore find that (i) the plaintiffs' injuries were capable of being caused by their repetitive work, (ii) those injuries were, in fact, caused by this particular work and (iii) that those injuries were foreseeable."

"On the evidence before me in this case it is clear that there was not a sophisticated or indeed any real programme of educating and warning employees."

"I would emphasise it is particularly important that the warning should contain an explanation of why it is necessary to report."

"It is clear from the evidence in this case that no warnings were given to the employees and in consequence the defendants were in breach of their duty to give the appropriate warnings and to enforce a proper sense of awareness of the dangers of contracting various work related upper limb disorders that the plaintiffs in these cases have in fact contracted."

TENOSYNOVITIS – A CASE OF MISTAKEN IDENTITY

ALEXANDER -v- H C C TINSLEY & SON
H H JUDGE LANGAN
NORWICH COUNTY COURT
15 OCTOBER 1991

The plaintiff failed to establish liability against the defendant because the judge found on the medical evidence that the plaintiff's carpal tunnel syndrome was not brought about by her work but was a naturally occurring spontaneous carpal tunnel syndrome in a lady in her middle years.

McSHERRY -v- BRITISH TELECOM PLC
LODGE -v- BRITISH TELECOM PLC
H H JUDGE JOHN BYRT Q C
MAYORS & CITY OF LONDON COURT
16 DECEMBER 1991

"In both cases, I have found that each plaintiff suffered RSI as a result of her work, the condition being brought about by a repetitive stereotype movement of unsupported arms and hands. Further, I have found that that strain has been substantially added to by the strains which arose from the working systems in place and poor posture due to poor ergonomics of the workstation, unsuitable chairs, and, in the case of Mrs Lodge, the uncorrected bad habits of the operator."

"... the crucial period during which the defendants' liability is to be determined is the year late 1981 to late 1982."

"On that totality of evidence, what would be the proper findings to make about the defendants' actual or constructive knowledge?"

"First, I am not satisfied that the defendants knew sufficient about the causal connection between RSI and keyboard work to warrant radical action in time to save either Mrs Lodge or Mrs McSherry, nor am I satisfied that they should be affected with constructive knowledge."

LITIGATION AND CASE LAW

"Between 1980 and 1984, there is a gap in the literature which specifically relates to RSI and keyboard work."

"I find that, having regard to the state of developing knowledge, there was insufficient scope in this instance for the defendants to come up with workable alterations in the systems in time to help the plaintiffs.

My next finding relates to liability concerning posture. I am satisfied that the defendants knew or ought to have known that postures of the sort adopted by Mrs McSherry and Mrs Lodge and their work colleagues were, in the course of time, likely to cause them serious musculo-skeletal injury. Accordingly, in my judgment, they were under continuing responsibility to ensure that those postures were corrected so as to mitigate, as best possible, the risk that the plaintiffs might suffer injury. In so finding, I consider it immaterial whether the bad posture was due to unsuitable chairs, the modesty panel or the operators' own choice of sitting position."

"I am satisfied that the defendants were in breach of their common law duty to the plaintiffs by reason of their failure to ensure correct posture was maintained."

"In this case, poor posture was only a contributive cause of the repetitive strain injuries suffered by the plaintiffs. The combination of intensive, repetitive keyboard work, carried out during shifts of prolonged periods of time, and poor posture was responsible for the full extent of the injuries these plaintiffs suffered. But, as I have already found, poor posture contributed substantially to those injuries and that, other things being equal, is sufficient to establish liability : see McGhee -v- National Coal Board (1972) 3 AER 1008.

Tenosynovitis – A Case Of Mistaken Identity

Further, it is sufficient in law if the tortfeasor should reasonably have foreseen that his breach of duty was likely to cause injury within the broad category of injury which was in fact caused : Hughes -v- Lord Advocate (1963) 1 AER 705. As I have found, I am satisfied that the defendants should have been aware that bad posture would cause musculo-skeletal problems. The fact that the injuries sustained were more extensive than those they might have envisaged is of no consequence in law.

In the result, I find the defendants liable in common law to the plaintiffs for the full extent of the pain and suffering they have experienced."

"... I am satisfied that, in both cases, the defendants failed to produce suitable chairs and that this amounted to a breach of their absolute duty under Section 14 of the Offices Shops & Railway Premises Act 1963. This breach of their obligation .... substantially contributed to the plaintiffs' injuries ...."

"... defendants were not to be imputed with knowledge, actual or constructive, that the keyboard work might cause RSI. It is therefore inappropriate that I should find the defendants in breach of duty by reason of their failure to warn the plaintiffs in this instance."

KELLY -v- BRITISH STEEL Plc
H H JUDGE FRICKER Q C
DONCASTER COUNTY COURT
22 JANUARY 1992

"I find that the plaintiff did suffer from what I call repetitive strain syndrome .... but that it was not just fatigue but a muscular strain."

"I find that tenosynovitis not proved."

Litigation And Case Law

"... it was not reasonably foreseeable that repetitive strain syndrome or this type of injury was likely or possible in any real sense from this work...".

"... it was not negligent at any stage for the employers to let this man, if he wished, continue his work involving radio controlled boxes, even though he was suffering some pain from repetitive strain factor."

"I find that the defendants took all reasonable precautions to protect the plaintiff by further re-adjustment or by allocation of work or otherwise and in all the circumstances the plaintiff's case fails."

Tenosynovitis – A Case Of Mistaken Identity

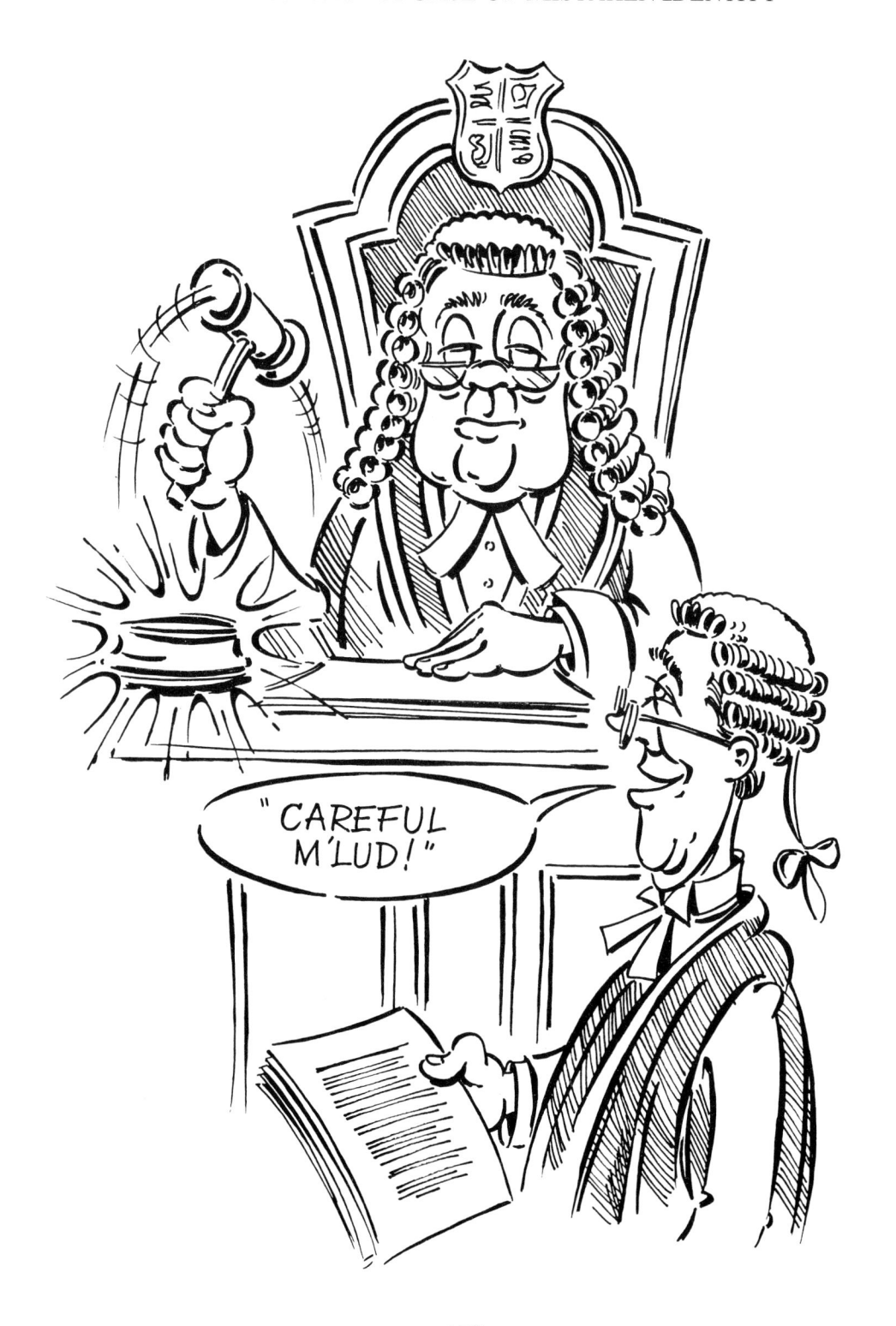

3. The Identifiable Legal Issues

By reference to the case law **the main legal issues** arising are identified and summarised.

1. The first question to be answered is whether or not the operation of which the claimant complains carries a foreseeable, inherent, specific and not insignificant risk of the claimant developing an ULD.

2. Should the above question be answered in the negative then in all probability the employers have a good defence to any claim brought. Should this question be answered in the affirmative, then the following points call for consideration:-
   (a) Have the employers discharged their duties to the claimant which arise in these circumstances?
   (b) Have the employers set out the work in a reasonable fashion eliminating all unnecessary sources of danger by applying proper ergonomic considerations?
   (c) Have the employers organised working conditions upon the same basis by instigating, for example, a rotation system and proper rest periods?
   (d) Have the employers instigated and operated a relatively sophisticated system of warnings both pre-employment in proper cases and post employment?
   (e) Are the physical problems from which the plaintiff suffered (which must be properly diagnosed) attributable to her employment and the matters of which she complains?

4. Damages : Examples of Court and other Awards

Awards of damages by the courts for this type of injury have been relatively few. The high sums featured by the headline writers are exceptional and usually related to the specific circumstances of the case.

Tenosynovitis – A Case Of Mistaken Identity

The following examples indicate levels of damages in decided cases:-

---
PRESLAND -v- G W PADLEY
1979

General damages £1,250 plus agreed special damages (unspecified). Plaintiff failed to satisfy court that continuing disability was causally connected.

BURGESS -v- THORN CONSUMER ELECTRONICS
1983

General damages £3,500 plus £7,531 loss of earnings and special damage. (No award for handicap on the labour market).

TREE & OTHERS -v- M K ELECTRONICS
1984

There were 5 consolidated actions:-

TREE — General damages £3,500 plus agreed special damages £764.41.

ECKERSLEY — General damages £750 plus agreed special damages £78.79.

DARVILLE — General damages £1,500 plus agreed special damages £229.15.

SOLLY — General damages £750 – no special damages.

BAKER — No award (causation not established).

Litigation And Case Law

PEPALL & OTHERS -v- THORN CONSUMER ELECTRONICS
1985

There were 10 consolidated actions:-

LIFE	General damages £1,500 (plus special damages for a period of 2 years).
HOUSTON	General damages £2,500 (plus special damages for a period of 18 months).
PENNICOTT	General damages £400 (plus special damages for a period of 5 months).
PEPALL	General damages of £5,000 (plus agreed special damages of £2,366.30).
RILEY	General damages £750 (plus agreed damages of £639.89).
YOUNG	General damages £2,250 – no special damages.
PRINCE	General damages £300 (plus special damages for a period of 6 months).
DAWKINS	General damages £400 (plus special damages for a period of 6 months).
EAMES	General damages £2,250 (plus agreed special damages of £7,633).
GORMAN	No award (causation not established) – general damages of £350 would have been awarded if case proven.

CAIRNS -v- PHILIPS ELECTRONICS LTD
1985

General damages £1,500 plus special damages of £3,100.

Tenosynovitis – A Case Of Mistaken Identity

GLEESON-BARTLETT -v- E B PACKERS
1990

Judgement for defendants but would have awarded £1,200 – no award for handicap on the open labour market.

NB *It is worth noting in GLEESON-BARTLETT that the court identified* **any** *assault on the wrist as a result of work ie inflammation, bruising, cuts, swelling or true tenosynovitis as giving an entitlement to damages* **excepting** *an injury so trivial or so much part of a day's work that it is right to treat it as de minimis.*

In the "other awards" category are awards of usually **agreed** figures (damages agreed between the parties rather than being awarded by the judge) and then simply **approved** by the court (usually an academic exercise).

The well known examples:-

BERNARD -v- MIDLAND BANK
1989

Agreed damages of £45,000 paid to a 30 year old secretary.

CARVER -v- WAVENEY APPLE GROWERS
1990

Agreed damages of £35,000 paid to an agricultural worker.

Litigation And Case Law

THE INLAND REVENUE CASES
1990

Agreed damages of £107,500 paid to three computer data clerks (visual display unit keyboard operators):-

Thomas	-	£42,500
Kay	-	£43,000
Armstrong	-	£22,000

PING & OTHERS -v- ESSELTE LETRASET LTD
1991

There were 9 consolidated actions:-

PING	Agreed general damages agreed special damages	£7,500.00 (plus £437.60)
DEADMAN	Agreed general damages agreed special damages	£6,000.00 (plus £461.65)
KING	Agreed general damages agreed special damages	£8,000.00 (plus £338.98)
GIBBS	Agreed general damages - special damages	£3,000.00 -
OAKS	Agreed general damages agreed special damages	£3,500.00 (plus £1,295.00)
ARCHER	Agreed general damages agreed special damages	£5,000.00 (plus £214.86)
MURTON	Agreed general damages agreed special damages	£5,500.00 (plus £262.48)
FERRARIS	Agreed general damages agreed special damages	£3,000.00 (plus £275.83)

Tenosynovitis – A Case Of Mistaken Identity

BEADLE General damages (not agreed) £3,000.00
(plus special damages £3,967.32
and four years future loss)

ALEXANDER -v- H C C TINSLEY & SONS
1991

Plaintiff failed to establish liability but would have been awarded general damages of £5,000 plus special damages of £400.

McSHERRY -v- BRITISH TELECOM PLC
LODGE -v- BRITISH TELECOM PLC
1991

General damages of £6,000 each plus special damages and interest to be agreed.

Other Guidance

Guidelines recently published by the Judicial Studies Board for the assessment of damages for personal injury cases render little assistance in relation to conditions for upper limb disorders. Tennis elbow is mentioned, other arm injuries classified as moderate or minor injuries attracting damages up to £5,000. Vibration white finger merits a section on its own covering three stages of injury due to prolonged vibration with a range of damages from £800 to the oddly precise figure of £4,875.

Litigation And Case Law

Other General Issues

1. An employer is under a duty to take reasonable care for the safety of his employees and he must not expose them to unnecessary risks.

2. The steps which an employer must take in order to fulfil the common law duty owed to his employees must be commensurate with the degree of risk involved and the potential gravity of the injury.

3. An employer must provide a safe system of work and safe plant and equipment whatever the risk involved.

4. Where for a particular employee the degree of risk is high and the potential gravity of the injury serious, an employer has a duty to prevent that employee from doing that work and if necessary to refuse to employ him/her.

5. Where the degree of risk and the potential gravity of the injury is low, the employer will fulfil his duty by informing the employee of the risks.

6. In assessing the standard of care required or in assessing what action is reasonable, it may be appropriate to look at the practice employed by other employers in the field.

7. Where an employee is abnormally susceptible, the employer should not be liable but he must expect some high degree of sensitivity within his workplace and take the appropriate precautions.

8. The occurrence of previous incidents is relevant in deciding whether an employer should have foreseen the likelihood of the incident in question. The absence however of such incidents does not justify an assumption by an employer that the system of work is safe.

9. If a danger is unknown at the time of the incident, the employer is **prima facie** not liable.

10. There is an imputation of knowledge to the employer if the danger is generally known.

11. It is the duty of the employer to acquire the degree of knowledge which is common in his particular trade.

Tenosynovitis – A Case Of Mistaken Identity

12. If the risk is unavoidable and inherent it is an **ordinary risk of service** against which the employer cannot be expected to protect his employees.

13. Employees have a duty to look to their own safety once they are apprised of a risk or hazard.

14. Usual considerations as to contributory negligence apply but should the employer be able to show that (all other things being equal) the plaintiff is unlikely to have acted upon warnings given, this might be a complete defence.

It is anticipated that emphasis on upper limb disorder will shift from factories to offices and for this reason it is important to consider what, in the absence hitherto of statutory regulations, the employer is deemed to know, and what is likely to come to the attention of the employer. There seems to be little if anything.

When confronted with claims in a new field it is logical to turn to legal text books. One of the leading text books on employers liability is, "Munkman's Employers' Liability". The 11th edition was published in 1990. Under the heading "Offices, Shops and Railway Premises" the following passage is found:-

> "In comparison with factories and mines, offices and shops are hardly a serious safety problem, apart from the insistence on fire precautions and safe floors and staircases, which is necessary everywhere. Workshops attached to shops and large stores are already subject to the Factories Act. Thus the welfare, rather than the safety requirements (lighting, ventilation, washing facilities) are the important things in shops and offices. Liability for breach of the safety sections is likely to arise mainly from falls on unsafe floors or stairs."

In these circumstances to prove that an injury has been caused by the employer's negligence it is necessary to show that he knew or ought to have known about the risk and could and should have done something about it. If this is the most a lawyer's text book can say about offices it is harsh to suggest that an employer should be saddled with greater knowledge.

Litigation And Case Law

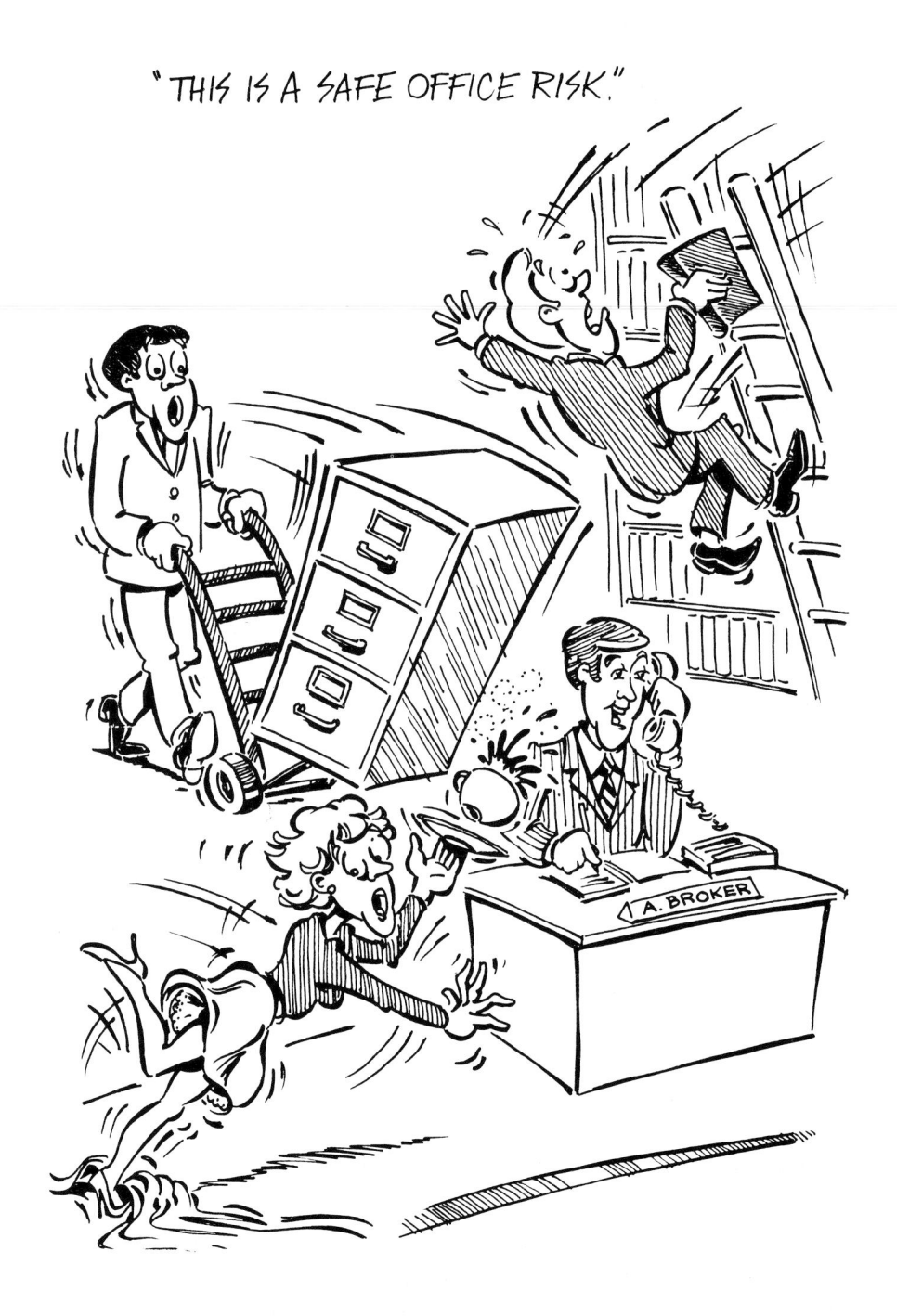

"THIS IS A SAFE OFFICE RISK."

ADVICE AND GUIDANCE TO EMPLOYERS

The susceptibility of the individual is very much a deciding factor in cases of upper limb disorder. Where it is not possible to predict who will suffer an injury doing this work, the fact that some do contract the condition does not necessarily make the employer liable.

The basic duty of the company to its employees is to provide a safe system of work and to take all reasonable steps to safeguard against injury in respect of risks of which the company knows or ought to know.

It is generally acknowledged that the principles to be applied are comprehensively set out in the Judgement of SWANWICK J. in STOKES -v- GKN (See page 121).

The risks of upper limb disorder arising from certain areas of industry have been known for many years. It is essential therefore that there should be in place a system that informs and warns employees and prospective employees of such risks and leads to the early identification and treatment of those affected.

A safe system of work with warnings to employees is required in order to comply with legal requirements. (A theme running strongly through all the case law referred to).

The widely differing conditions that exist in many areas of industry and in the commercial sector suggest that advice and guidance may only be offered on a very broad, general basis. Such guidance may not be sufficiently precise to deal with every situation arising at every firm but may be used as the basis of a health and safety policy that can be adapted to individual needs.

There is clearly a worry among some employers that a system introduced along these lines may bring the condition to the attention of the workforce. The alternative however is to take no action at all which may result at some stage in the future in more workers being injured followed by claims with lesser prospects of a successful defence.

ADVICE AND GUIDANCE TO EMPLOYERS

As part of a preventative strategy a formal policy on upper limb disorder should be established and employees made aware of its existence. This involves elements of risk assessment and planning.

Where a particular job or range of jobs is suspect, some form of risk assessment should be made to identify the specific risk factors. Where risk assessment is likely to be complex, expert help should be sought.

If an expert's report is obtained, full and proper consideration must be given to implementing any recommendations made as a failure to do so without good reason may well have a detrimental effect on prevention and defence of future actions. It should be remembered that all reports obtained and any minutes relating to a consideration of the consultant's recommendations will be disclosable in any future legal actions.

It is recommended that consideration is given to the following areas as the starting point of a formal health and safety policy on upper limb disorder. Essentially the situation requires a common sense approach.

- Employers should be alert to reports and complaints of pain or discomfort in the upper limbs and steps must be taken to investigate and monitor such complaints.
- The nature of the complaint should be established.
- The company must review the practices of a department where upper limb complaints have arisen and in consultation with medical advisers investigate **possible** avenues with a view to reducing the potential risk to employees.
- Ideally where a problem is known or suspected, the employee should be taken from the cause and put onto alternative work.
- The position thereafter should be reviewed in the light of medical evidence.
- In considering the precautions where nothing physical can be achieved (even with work rotation a susceptible individual may still develop symptoms), it is essential that the employee must at all times be kept informed and allowed a choice between **accepting a** potential risk and leaving the job.
- Having regard to the type of industry involved, a company may have greater than average knowledge of the risks and may therefore be obliged to take more than the average or standard precautions.

Tenosynovitis – A Case Of Mistaken Identity

- Once it is established that there is an **incidence** of this type of condition (knowledge), the employer is obliged to review the system of work to consider whether it can be altered to reduce the potential hazard either by:-

    1. Reduction or curtailment of the process.
    2. Mechanisation.
    3. Rotation.

- Having reviewed the system and considered and implemented any possible alterations the conclusion may be that the **fundamental** system cannot be altered.
- The legal duty upon the employer in these circumstances is that those employees at risk from the process or occupation must be **warned** that some employees may have a **predisposition** to this type of condition and doing this work may bring about such a condition.
- Employees must be told that if they have any hand, arm or wrist problem they should immediately advise their manager, personnel manager, supervisor, works doctor or nurse.
- Ideally the worker affected should be removed from the work temporarily pending examination by the company doctor.
- Where there is no permanent or visiting company doctor, the employee must be referred to his or her own general practitioner.
- The examining doctor should be encouraged to make a precise diagnosis and to suggest the best option available to the employer:-

    1. If it is a minor problem of a temporary nature unlikely to recur, whether there is a reasonable possibility of the employee returning to normal duties with no further ill effects.
    2. If it is a more serious problem with possible long term effects, whether the employer should:-
        - consider a temporary transfer to alternative employment
        - consider a permanent transfer to alternative employment
        - terminate the employment.

- If the condition is alleviated by a **temporary transfer** of employment,

ADVICE AND GUIDANCE TO EMPLOYERS

  then after a suitable period of time the employee may be returned to the original occupation suitably monitored to ensure there is no recurrence.
- If there is no recurrence there is no reason why the employee should not continue.
- If there is a recurrence then it would seem apparent that the employee is unsuited for the work available.
- In that event **permanent transfer** to suitable employment of a lighter nature must be considered but if not available then ultimately the employee must on medical grounds be advised to obtain **alternative employment** elsewhere. However where there is only a minimal risk of minimal injury the employee may elect to accept the risk.
- The employer must ensure that any alternative employment offered is suitable in all respects, including medical. Should the employee refuse reasonable alternative employment or is not prepared to accept the minimal risk then the only option left may be to terminate the employment.
- In view of the possible potential in lost earnings to the employee, termination of employment should be taken as a final option only after exhaustive enquiry.
- There will be occasions when employees should be removed from the process even if this means cessation of employment.
- **The employer should ensure that at every stage careful records are maintained of induction and training courses, general and specific warnings and advice.**
- Although there is no duty upon an employer to warn **prospective** employees of the risk of ULD, it not being known at that stage what work the prospective employees may be doing, nevertheless, where appropriate, employers are encouraged to warn potential employees of any known risk before they commence employment.
- Once it is clear that certain jobs may provoke this type of condition then it is advisable to alert all new starters, both at the **initial interview** and when the **offer of employment** is made that some individuals may be susceptible to hand and arm problems and in that event that they should immediately bring them to the employer's attention

Tenosynovitis – A Case Of Mistaken Identity

(pre-employment warning).

- All letters offering employment should where appropriate contain a specific advice and warning of this nature; alternatively it may be covered by a contract of employment.
- Employees must be provided with **essential details** of the likely symptoms and medical conditions that may occur. It must be made clear that continued working whilst suffering from such symptoms can cause permanent damage.
- It may also be advisable to obtain a completed Declaration of Health before allowing the prospective employee to commence employment to include a question whether the prospective employee suffers or has suffered from upper limb disorder or hand and arm related complaints.
- Such declaration could incorporate **warning and advice** along the following lines:-

> "In this industry work often involves force or rapid and repetitive movement of the hands. This can give rise to aching and discomfort – a condition sometimes known as tenosynovitis or a like condition which occasionally leads to a period of temporary or even permanent disability. This is likely to occur most often with new employees, personnel returning to work after absence or those involved in a change of process.
>
> Should you at any time experience any aching and discomfort in the arms, wrists or hands which may be related to your working environment, you are under a duty to report such symptoms promptly to your Supervisor/Works Nurse/Medical Centre etc who will take appropriate steps in an endeavour to overcome them.
>
> You will be kept advised of any developments following your reporting action."

ADVICE AND GUIDANCE TO EMPLOYERS

An acknowledgement that such advice and warning is understood is desirable.

- Additionally consideration should be given to posting similar advice at various sites such as works notice boards, canteens and changing rooms to ensure that employees are reminded where appropriate of the risks on a daily basis.
- Warnings of this nature should be repeated when and wherever possible.
- Alternatively prospective employees may be given appropriate warning by means of a separate written notice for which a signed receipt should be obtained.
- There is a duty upon the employer to warn and **to continue to warn** where a person is put on work that involves **inherent specific and not insignificant risk** of developing ULD's.
- It follows that **warning** by way of an **explanation** of the risk must be accompanied by **regular education** emphasising the particular steps which could be taken to reduce the risk.
- Warnings must not be confined to prospective employees. Similar criteria apply to **existing employees** where there is a **foreseeable or known risk** of injury and accordingly steps must be taken to inform or warn existing employees.
- **Compliance with the new Regulations which apply to visual display screens and workstations is essential.**
- **We advocate consultation and co-operation with employees either directly or through a staff association or union to combat this and other health related problems. The first priority for all should be one of prevention rather than compensation. Unlike some diseases, say noise induced hearing loss, upper limb disorders are neither insidious in onset nor untreatable and progression to a severe condition is rare and usually only results from ignoring the early symptoms.**

RESEARCH PUBLICATIONS/ REFERENCES

Date of Publication	Author(s)	Publication	Title
1907	**Departmental Committee on Compensation for Industrial Diseases**	HMSO	Report of the Departmental Committee on Compensation for Industrial Diseases
1918	**Secretary of State**	S R & O No 287	Extension to Workmen's (Compensation Act 1906)
1929	**Secretary of State**	S R & O No 2	Extension to Workmen's (Compensation Act 1925)
Sep 1931	**H R Conn**	Ohio State Medical Journal	Tenosynovitis
Apr 1937	**N J Howard**	The Journal of Bone & Joint Surgery	Peritendinitis Crepitans
1948	**Minister of National Insurance**	S I 1948 No 1371	The National Insurance (Industrial Injuries) (Prescribed Diseases) Regulations 1948
1950	**Minister of National Insurance**	HMSO	Notes on the Diagnosis of Occupational Diseases
1951	**A R Thompson L W Plewes E G Shaw**	British Journal of Industrial Medicine	Peritendinitis Crepitans & Simple Tenosynovitis – a Clinical Study of 544 cases in Industry
1951	**J A Smiley**	British Journal of Industrial Medicine	The Hazards of Ropemaking
1955	**D Hunter**	English Universities Press	The Diseases of Occupations
1956	**R N Wilson S Wilson**	The Practitioner	Tenosynovitis in Industry

Research Publications/References

Date of Publication	Author(s)	Publication	Title
Apr 1958	**Industrial Injuries Advisory Council**	Command 416	Review of the Prescribed Diseases Schedule
1958	**Minister of Pensions & National Insurance**	S I 1958 No 1068	The National Insurance (Industrial Injuries) (Prescribed Diseases) Amendment Regulations
1959	**P R Lipscomb**	CLIN. ORTH 13	Tenosynovitis of the Hand & Wrist, Carpal Tunnel Syndrome, de Quervain's Disease, Trigger Digit
1965	**H M Chief Inspector of Factories**	HMSO	Annual Report of H M Chief Inspector of Factories on Industrial Health
Nov 1965	**T A Lamphier**	Industrial Medicine & Surgery	De Quervain's Disease
Nov 1966	**L Hymovich M Lindholm**	Journal of Occupational Medicine	Hand, Wrist & Forearm Injuries
1969	**D Hunter**	English Universities Press	The Diseases of Occupations
1970	**H M Chief Inspector of Factories**	HMSO	Annual Report of H M Chief Inspector of Factories
1971	**J T Watkins**	International Labour Office	Encyclopaedia of Occupational Health
1972	**DHSS**	HMSO	Notes on the Diagnosis of Occupational Diseases
Oct 1972	**R Welch**	Industrial Medicine	The Causes of Tenosynovitis in Industry
Nov 1972	**Department of Employment**	Employment Medical Advisers Notes of Guidance	Beat Conditions, Tenosynovitis
1973	**R Welch**	Ergonomics	The Measurement of Physiological Predisposition to Tenosynovitis
1976	**S S Guirguis**	Occupational Health in Ontario	Tenosynovitis

TENOSYNOVITIS – A CASE OF MISTAKEN IDENTITY

Date of Publication	Author(s)	Publication	Title
Sep 1977	**Health & Safety Executive**	Guidance Note MS.10	Beat Conditions, Tenosynovitis
Nov 1977	**J G P Williams**	The Journal of Bone & Joint Surgery	Surgical Management of Traumatic Non-Infective **Tenosynovitis of the** Wrist Extensors
Jul 1979	**T J Armstrong D B Chaffin**	Journal of Occupational Medicine	Carpal Tunnel Syndrome & Selected Personal Attributes
1980	**C Mackay**	Health & Safety Executive Research Paper 10	Human Factors Aspects of Visual Display Unit Operation
1980	**D Hunter**	English Universities Press	The Diseases of Occupations
Dec 1980	**K Maeda W Hunting E Grandjean**	Journal of Occupational Medicine	Localised Fatigue in Accounting Machine Operators
1982	**R Welch**	International Labour Office	Encyclopaedia of Occupational Health
Feb 1982	**T J Armstrong & Others**	Journal of the American Industrial Hygiene Association	Investigation of Cumulative Trauma Disorders in a Poultry Processing Plant
Jul 1982		Workers Health Centre	Tenosynovitis & Other Occupational Over-Use Injuries
Aug 1982	**J Mathews N Calabrese**	Australian Council of Trade Unions Health & Safety Bulletin	Guide-lines for the Prevention of Repetitive Strain Injury Injury
Oct 1982		The Lancet	Writers' Cramp
Dec 1982	**J Anderson**	Safety Management	Rheumatic Diseases
1983	**DHSS**	HMSO	Notes on the Diagnosis of Occupational Diseases
1983	**Health & Safety Executive**	HMSO	Visual Display Units
1983	**R Welch**	International Labour Office	Encyclopaedia of Occupational Health & Safety

Research Publications/References

Date of Publication	Author(s)	Publication	Title
Aug 1984		Bulletin of the Queensland Workers Health Centre	Over-Use Injuries
1985	**GMBATU**	College Hill Press	Tackling Teno : A GMB Guide to Tenoysynovitis & Repetitive Strain Injury
Apr 1985		Workers Health Centre	Over-Use Injuries
Jul 1985	**N M Hadler**	The Journal of Hand Surgery	Illness in the Workplace: The Challenge of Musculo-Skeletal Symptoms
Oct 1985	**K Johnson**	Professional Safety	Analytical Report on the Causes & Preventions of Carpal Tunnel Syndrome
1986	**P W Buckle**	Contemporary Ergonomics	Ergonomic Aspects of Tenosynovitis & Carpal Tunnel Syndrome in Production Line Workers
Jan 1986	**S Eckles**	Environmental Health	Repetition Strain Injury - Keyboard Operators Disease
Jan 1986	**S Collier**	Health & Safety at Work	Tackling Teno
Jan 1986	**G Bammer & Others**	Research School of Social Sciences Australian National University	ANU Research on RSI
Jun 1986	**C Semple**	The Journal of Hand Surgery	Tenosynovitis
Nov 1986	**D Ross**	Occupational Health & Safety	Dupuytren's Contracture
1987	**H A Waldron**	British Journal of Industrial Medicine	Anyone for Teno?
1987	**B A Silverstein L J Fine T J Armstrong**	American Journal of Industrial Medicine	Occupational Factors & Carpal Tunnel Syndrome
1987	**D S Chatterjee**	Journal of the Society of Occupational Medicine	Repetition Strain Injury - a Recent Review

Tenosynovitis – A Case Of Mistaken Identity

Date of Publication	Author(s)	Publication	Title
Feb 1987	**G Bammer**	Health & Safety at Work	Repetition Strain Injuries Affect VDU Operators Too
Apr 1987	**J L Kearns**	Occupational Health Review	Tenosynovitis
Jun 1987	**G Evans**	British Medical Journal	Tenosynovitis in Industry: Menace or Misnomer
Sep 1987	**T J Armstrong**	The Journal of Hand Surgery	Ergonomics Considerations in Hand & Wrist Tendinitis
Sep 1987		Health & Safety Information Bulletin	Draft BSI Standard on VDU Ergonomics
1987	**D Hunter**	English Universities Press	The Diseases of Occupations
Jan 1988		London Hazard Centre Trust	Repetition Strain Injuries
Feb 1988	**D C R Ireland**	The Journal of Hand Surgery	Psychological & Physical Aspects of Occupational Arm Pain
Mar 1988	**S Ross**	Occupational Health & Safety	Tenosynovitis
Oct 1988	**S Fournier**	The Canadian Centre for Occupational Health & Safety	RSI & The Causality Issue
1988	**V Putz-Anderson**	Taylor & Francis	Cumulative Trauma Disorders
Jan 1989	**C J English & Others**	Institute of Occupational Medicine	Clinical Epidemiological Study of Relations Between Upper Limb Soft Tissue Disorders & Repetitive Movement at Work
Jan 1989	**H A Bird**	Arthritis & Rheumatism Council	Work-Related Syndromes
Feb 1989		Occupational Health	How to Recognise RSI
Jun 1989	**R A Green C A Briggs**	Journal of Occupational Medicine	Effect of Over-Use Injury and the Importance of Training on the Use of Adjustable Workstations by Keyboard Operators
Aug 1989	**N Barton**	British Medical Journal	Repetitive Strain Disorder

Research Publications/References

Date of Publication	Author(s)	Publication	Title
Sep 1989	**C J English**	The Practitioner	Repetitive Strain Injuries
1990	**D Thompson & Others**	The University of Birmingham	Occurrence & Mechanism of Occupational Repetitive Strain Injury
1990		The RSI Association	Help & Information for those who suffer from Repetitive Strain Injury
Jun 1990		Official Journal of the European Communities	Council Directive on the Minimum Safety & Health Requirements for Work with Display Screen Equipment
Aug 1990		Health & Safety Information Bulletin	Medical & Legal Aspects of Upper Limb Disorders
Sep 1990		Health & Safety Information Bulletin	Preventing & Managing Upper Limb Disorders
Oct 1990	**Health & Safety Executive**	HMSO	Work Related Upper Limb Disorders – A Guide to Prevention
Dec 1990	**R J Graves**	The Health & Safety Practitioner	Repetition Strain Injury
Mar 1991	**A Nicholson**	Health & Safety at Work	Out on a Limb

APPENDIX

Employers requiring more detailed information and professional advice on the ergonomic aspects of work related upper limb disorder should consult a qualified ergonomist or an institute such as a university department specialising in this field.

The Ergonomics Society has a list of members who have experience in preventing work related upper limb disorders. They have recognised qualifications and as members of its professional register are required to abide by its professional code of conduct.

The list of members is available to anyone wishing to contact the Society.

The Society also publishes its register of professional ergonomists.

Contact

Central Office, The Ergonomics Society

University of Technology, Devonshire House, Devonshire Square, Loughborough, Leicester, LE11 3DW
Tel. 0509 234904

Other useful organisations include the following:-

Ergonomics Research Unit

Robens Institute of Health & Safety, University of Surrey, Guildford, Surrey, GU2 5XH
Tel 0483 509203

The Unit carries out research, runs training courses and conferences and provides an ergonomics consultancy service.

Appendix

Health & Safety Executive
Health Policy Division, Baynards House, 1 Chepstow Place, Westbourne Grove, London W2 4TF
Tel 071 243 6000

The HSE has published a number of guidance documents on WRULD's and VDU's.

HUSAT Research Institute
University of Technology, The Elms, Elms Grove, Loughborough, Leicestershire, LE11 1RG
Tel 0509 611088

Provides consultancy and training services on the management and prevention of upper limb disorder amongst keyboard operators.

Ergonomics Training Centre Ltd
Suite 9, Museum House, Museum Street, London WC1A 1JT
Tel 071 636 5912

Provides ergonomics skills training courses and consultancy on workplace ergonomics.

Ice Ergonomics Ltd
75 Swingbridge Road, Loughborough, Leicestershire, LE11 0JB
Tel 0509 236161

Industrial Ergonomics Group and Ergonomics Information Analysis Centre
School of Manufacturing and Mechanical Engineering, The University of Birmingham, Birmingham B15 2TT
Tel 021 414 4239

Institute of Occupational Medicine Ltd
8 Roxburgh Place, Edinburgh, EH8 9SU
Tel 031 667 5131

INDEX

abduction 24
abductor pollicis longus 56, 66
addresses 160-61
adduction 24
advice 11, 148-53
age 51
air quality 70, 76
ALEXANDER -V- H C C TINSLEY & SON 134, 144
alternative employment 151
analgesics 74
anti-depressants 74
anti-inflammatory drugs 74
arms, *see* upper limb disorders; upper limbs
Australia 20, 23, 48-9
automation 33, 98
awards of damages 139-44
   guidelines 144

beat conditions 92-3
BERNARD -V- MIDLAND BANK 142
biomechanical factors 70
bones 38-9
bricklaying 90
Bridge, John C 11
BURGESS -V- THORN CONSUMER ELECTRONICS 83-4, 116, 125
   damages 140

CAIRNS -V- PHILIPS ELECTRONICS LTD 141
carpal tunnel 25
carpal tunnel syndrome 36, 54-6, 92

ALEXANDER -V- H C C TINSLEY & SON 134
carpus 40, 41
cartilage 25
cartilaginous joints 38
CARVER -V- WAVENEY APPLE GROWERS 142
case law 121-137, *see also* litigation, individual cases listed alphabetically
causation 109-11, 113
CBI (Confederation Of British Industry) 103
cellulite peritendineuse 66
cervical - (prefix) 25
chicken preparing 31, 32, 33, 94
   LANE -V- SUN VALLEY POULTRY 83, 126-7
chuck grip 25
claims 15
   awards of damages 139-44
      guidelines 144
   causation and medical evidence 109-11
   handling 113-17
   incorrect diagnosis 16-17
   injury and disablement benefit 34-5
   investigation 109
   liability 111-12
   record of action taken 117-19
   summary of evidence 117-19
clavicle 39
clinical diagnosis, *see* diagnosis
clinical features 51-2

compensation claims 15, 49
   awards of damages 139-44

INDEX

guidelines 144
causation and medical evidence 109-11
handling 113-17
incorrect diagnosis 16-17
investigation 109
liability 111-12
record of action taken 117-19
summary of evidence 117-19
computers, *see* keyboard operators; visual display units
concentration 48
cortisone 64, 65, 74
costs 15
Cox, Professor Tom 78
cramp 47, 61, 93, 94
prescribed diseases 86-8, 91
crepitans 27
crepitus 25, 66
cumulative trauma disorder 23
cuneiform bone 41

damages 139-44
guidelines 144
De Quervain's Disease 56-8
deafness 131
degenerative joint disease 68
delayed reporting 72
dermatitis 83, 122
dexterity 43-4
diagnosis 25, 52, 98
incorrect 16-17, 72
disablement benefit 35
discomfort, *see* pain
display screens 78-9, 102-8, *see also* keyboard operators
dorsiflexion 25
DSS Regulations 17
prescribed diseases 34, 36
duty of care 120-21, 145-6
dysfunction 25

elbow 40, 53
epicondylitis 25, 64-5

pronator teres syndrome 68
employers
advice and guidance 11, 148-53
claims against, *see* claims
cost of claims 15
duty of care 12-21, 145-6
knowledge and warning 82-4
liability 111-12
liability insurance 11-12
personnel services 72, 79-81
statutory duty, *see* statutory duty
engineering controls 75-8
expert evidence 115
epi- (prefix) 25
epicondylitis 25, 64-5
equipment design 76
ergonomics 10, 11, 49, 75-8, 98
Ergonomics Society 160
European Community 100, 102-3
evidence 109-11, 115, 116
summary 117-19
expert evidence 115
extension 25
extensor pollicis brevis 56, 66
extensor retinaculum 55
extensor tenosynovitis 62
eye strain 70, 77, 106

Factories Act 1833 10
Factories Act 1961 100, 116
factory work 9-10, 31, 94
fatigue 21, 47, 48, 66-7, 98
fibrous joints 38
fingers 40, 43, 44
Dupuytren's Contracture 58-9
tenosynovitis 62, 63
trigger finger 63-4
Finkelstein's Test 26
flexion 26
flexor retinaculum 43, 55
flexor tenosynovitis 55, 56, 62
force 19, 46, 70
forearm 43, 44, 53

epicondylitis 64-5
occupational cramp 61
peritendinitis crepitans 66-7
prescribed diseases 91-2
pronator teres syndrome 68
radial tunnel syndrome 68
tenosynovitis 62, 63
foreseeability 116
FOX -v- CHAMPION SPARKING PLUG CO
   LTD 132-3
frozen shoulder 68
functional disability 52

Gamekeeper's Thumb 59
ganglion 59
gender 51
   carpal tunnel syndrome 56
   De Quervain's Disease 58
   trigger finger and thumb 63
general practitioners 16
GLEESON-BARTLETT -v- E B PACKERS
   131
   damages 142
golfers' elbow 64
grasp and pinch 43, 57
grip 43, 44, 52, 57, 62
Guidance Notes 92-5
   1990 95-6

hand 43-4, 53
   carpal tunnel syndrome 54-6
   De Quervain's Disease 56-8
   Dupuytren's Contracture 58-9
   Gamekeepers' Thumb 59
   occupational cramp 61
   prescribed diseases 87-8, 89, 91-2
   tenosynovitis 62
   trigger finger and thumb 63-4
Heath and Safety at Work etc. Act 1974
   95, 100, 102
Health and Safety (Display Screen
   Equipment) Regulations 1992 102-8

Health and Safety Executive 11, 14, 23
   address 161
   carpal tunnel syndrome 55
   Guidance Notes 92-5
      1990 95-6
   musculo-skeletal disease 35
   visual display units (VDU's) 78-9, 103
hearing loss 15, 131
heating 70, 76
historical outline 9-11
housework 56, 70
Howard N J 66
HUGHES -v- LORD ADVOCATE 136
humerus 39, 40
   epicondylitis 64
humidity 70, 76
hydrocortisone 64, 65, 74

immobilisation 74
induction training 81, 151
Industrial Injuries Advisory Council 36,
   88, 92
Industrial Injuries Scheme 34
inflammation 46
   epicondylitis 64
   tenosynovitis 62-3
information 11
   visual display units (VDU's) 106-7
injections 64, 65, 74
injury 46
injury benefit 34
Inland Revenue cases 143
insurance companies
   advice and guidance 11
   claims handling 113
Ireland, D C R 48, 49
Iron Trades Employers Insurance
   Association Limited 15

Japan 23
job rotation 71, 79

INDEX

joints 38-9
  elbow 40
  hand 43-4
  pathology 47
  shoulder 39
  wrist 40-41
JOSEPH -v- MINISTRY OF DEFENCE 83
Judicial Studies Board 144

KELLY -v- BRITISH STEEL PLC 136-7
keyboard operators 134-6, *see also* visual display units
KOSSINSKI -v- CHRYSLER (UK) LTD 122

Labour Force Survey 1990 35-6
LANE -v- SUN VALLEY POULTRY 83, 126-7
LAWLER -v- IMI YORKSHIRE COPPER TUBE LTD 131-2
legislation, *see* statutory duty
leisure activities 70
liability 111-12, 114
liability insurance 11-12
ligaments 26, 39, 40, 41
  flexor retinaculum 43
litigation 120, *see also* case law
  awards of damages 139-44
    guidelines 144
  conduct of the reasonable and prudent employer 120-121
  identifiable legal issues 139
LODGE -v- BRITISH TELECOM PLC 134-6
  damages 144
lunate bone 41

Mackay, Colin 48
Management of Health and Safety at Work Regulations 1992 100-102
manual capacity 43-4
McGHEE -v- NATIONAL COAL BOARD 135
McSHERRY -v- BRITISH TELECOM PLC 108, 134-6
  damages 144
mechanisation 33, 98
median nerve 44
  carpal tunnel syndrome 54, 55
medical discharge 116
medical evidence 109-11
metacarpal neck 63, 64
metacarpals 40
mining 86, 93
monotony 48
mood 48
MUNKMAN'S EMPLOYERS' LIABILITY 146
muscles 39, 40, 43
  epicondylitis 64-5
  fatigue 21, 66-7
  pathology 47
  peritendinitis crepitans 66-7
musculo-skeletal disease 22, 35, 36

National Insurance (Industrial Injuries) (Prescribed Diseases) Amendment Regulations 1958 90
National Insurance (Industrial Injuries) (Prescribed Diseases) Regulations 1948 87
neck 53, 68
negligence, *see* duty of care; risk reduction
NELSON -v- PLESSEY 123
nerve supply 43-4
noise 15, 70
numbness 52, 68
  carpal tunnel syndrome 55

occupational cervicobrachial disorder 23
occupational cramp 61, 91, 93, 94
occupational disabilities 10, 30-33
  Labour Force Survey 1990 35-6
  prescribed diseases 86-92
occupational health 11
occupational risk factors 69
  biomechanical factors 70

Tenosynovitis – A Case Of Mistaken Identity

unsafe systems of work   71-2
oedema   46
Offices Shops and Railway Premises Act 1963   136
official guidance   92-5
   1990   95-6
over-use injury   22

pain   47, 51-2
   carpal tunnel syndrome   55
   De Quervain's Disease   57
   peritendinitis crepitans   66
palmar fascia   58
palmar flexion   26
paraesthesia   26, 52
pathology   46-7
PEPALL & OTHERS -V- THORN CONSUMER ELECTRONICS   82-3, 84, 127-8
   damages   141
peri- (prefix)   27
periarthritis   27
peritendinitis   27
peritendinitis crepitans   62, 63
personnel services   72, 79-81
phalanges   40
Phalens Test   27
physiotherapy   74
PING & OTHERS -V- ESSELTE LETRASET LTD   133
   damages   143-4
posture   10, 70, 76
   repetitive strain injury   134-5
   static loading   19-20, 46, 47
prescribed diseases   34, 36, 86-92
PRESLAND -V- G W PADLEY LTD   82, 123
   damages   140
prevention   74, 149
   competent personnel function   79-81
   engineering controls and ergonomic factors   75-8
   knowledge and warning   82-4
prevention *continued*
   organisation of works systems   78-9

risk assessment and planning   84-5
pronation   27
pronator teres syndrome   68
psychosocial stress   48-9, 98

radial nerve   44
radial styloid   56, 57, 66
radial tunnel syndrome   68
radius   40
Ramazzini, Bernardino   10
records   117-19, 151
repetitive activities   15, 19-20, 46-7, 70
   psychosocial stress   48
repetitive strain injuries (RSI's)   14, 48-9
   case law   134-6
   definition   20-22
      medically imprecise   23
   occupational incidence   33-4
   upper limb, *see* upper limb disorders
research publications   154-9
rest   73-4
retinaculum   54-5
reversible fatigue syndrome   23
rheumatoid arthritis   68
ribs   39
risk reduction   74, 149, *see also* duty of care
   assessment and planning   84-5
   competent personnel function   79-81
   engineering controls and ergonomic factors   75-8
   knowledge and warning   82-4
   organisation of works systems   78-9
Robens Institute   55
rotator cuff tendinitis   68

scaphoid bone   41
scapula   39
self employed persons   35
sensation   43-4
sheaths (tendons)   46, 54
   De Quervain's Disease   57, 58

INDEX

prescribed diseases   87-8, 89, 91-2
   traumatic tenosynovitis   62
   trigger finger and thumb   63-4
shoulder   39, 53, 68
Social Security Act 1975   92
spondylitis   68
sporting activities   70
sprains   27, 46
static loading   19-20, 46, 47, 70
statistics (prescribed tenosynovitis)   16, 34
statutory duty
   Factories Act 1961   100
   Health and Safety at Work etc Act 1974   100, 102
   Health and Safety (Display Screen Equipment) Regulations 1992   102-8
   Management of Health and Safety at Work Regulations 1992   100-102
Statutory Sick Pay   35
stenosing tenosynovitis crepitans   63-4
stenosis   28, 56-7
stiffness   52
STOKES -v- GUEST, KEEN & NETTLEFORD (BOLTS & NUTS) LTD   121, 148
strains   28, 46
stress   46, 47
   mechanical   70, 76
   psychosocial   48-9
supervision   71
supination   28
supraspinatous tendinitis   68
surgery   58, 59, 64, 74
Swanwick J   121, 148
Sweden   23
swelling   52
   carpal tunnel syndrome   56
   ganglion   59
   peritendinitis crepitans   66
symptoms   51-2
   delayed reporting   72
   early reporting   80
   record of action taken   117-19, 151
symptoms *continued*
   reporting and claims handling   115-16

synovial joints   38-9
synovial membrane   28
synovitis   28, 87-8, 89

tactile sensation   43
task variation   71, 79
telegraphists' cramp   86, 87, 88
temperature   70, 76
tendons   28, 39, 40, 41, 43, 44
   carpal tunnel syndrome   54-5
   De Quervain's Disease   56-8
   pathology   46, 47
   peritendinitis crepitans   66-7
   prescribed diseases   87-8, 89, 91-2
   shoulder and neck   68
   traumatic inflammation   62-3
   trigger finger and thumb   63-4
tendovaginitis   28
tennis elbow   17, 64, 90, 144
teno- (prefix)   28
tenosynovitis   62-63, *see also* upper limb disorders
   case law, *see* case law
   definition   14, 22, 28
   duty to warn   83
   extensor   62
   flexor   55, 56, 62
   incidence in occupational categories   31-3
   incorrect diagnosis   16-17, 66, 67, 98
   official guidance   92-5
   statistics   16, 34
   stenosing   56, 58
Thackrah, Dr Charles Turner   10
thermal environment   70, 76
Thompson, A R and Plewes, L W   67
thoracic outlet syndrome   68
thumb   43, 44
   De Quervain's Disease   56-8
   Gamekeepers' Thumb   59
   tenosynovitis   63
thumb *continued*
   trigger thumb   63-4

tingling   52, 68
trades unions   11, 18, 49
training   81, 151
  visual display units (VDU's)   106
trauma   70
traumatic tenosynovitis   62-3
treatment   73-4
TREE & OTHERS -v- MK ELECTRICS   125-6
  damages   140
Triquetrum   41
TUC (Trades Union Congress)   103
twisters' cramp   86, 87, 88
typing   15

ulna   40
ulnar nerve   40, 44
United States   23
upper limb disorders
  carpal tunnel syndrome   54-6
  case law, *see* case law
  clinical diagnosis   52, 98
  clinical features   51-2
  compensation, *see* compensation claims
  De Quervain's Disease   56-8
  definitions   14, 23, 98
  description of complaint   53-4
  Dupuytren's Contracture   58-9
  employers' responsibilities, *see* employers
  epicondylitis   64-5
  Gamekeepers' Thumb   59
  ganglion   59
  incidence   98
    claims for injury and disablement benefit   34-5
    occupational categories   30-33
  incorrect diagnosis   16-17
  increased reporting   18
  litigation, *see* litigation
  occupational cramp   61

  occupational risk factors   69
  biomechanical factors   70
  unsafe systems of work   71-2
  official guidance   92-5
    1990   95-6
  pathology   46-7
  peritendinitis crepitans   66-7
  prescribed diseases   34, 36, 86-92
  prevention and risk reduction   74, 99
    competent personnel function   79-81
    engineering controls and ergonomic factors   75-8
    knowledge and warning   82-4
    organisation of works systems   78-9
    risk assessment and planning   84-5
  pronator teres syndrome   68
  psychosocial factors   48-9
  radial tunnel syndrome   68
  repetitive activities   15
  research publications/references   154-9
  shoulder and neck   68
  tenosynovitis   62-3
  treatment   73-4
  trigger finger and thumb   63-4
upper limb strain injury (ULSI)   22
upper limbs
  elbow   40
  hand   43-4
  shoulder   39
  structure and function   38-9
  wrist   40-41
USA   23

vibration   70, 77-8
vibration white finger   15, 83, 124, 144
visual display units (VDU's)   78-9, 102-8, *see also* keyboard operators
visual environment   70, 77

warnings   82-4, 115, 150, 152-3
  case law, *see* case law
weakness   52
WHITE -v- HOLBROOK PRECISION

INDEX

CASTINGS   83, 124
WHITNALL -V- CULROSE FOODS   129-30
WITHERS -V- PERRY CHAIN   83, 122
witnesses   116, 117
women
   carpal tunnel syndrome   56
   De Quervain's Disease   58
   trigger finger and thumb   63
work rate   71
Workmen's Compensation Act 1906   86
workplace environment   13, 150
   biomechanical factors   70
   design   75-6
   organisation of works systems   78-9
   unsafe systems of work   71-2
workstations   104-5
   repetitive strain injury   134-6
wrist   16, 40-41, 43, 44, 53
   carpal tunnel syndrome   54-6
   De Quervain's Disease   56-8
   epicondylitis   64, 65
   ganglion   59
   peritendinitis   66-7
   prescribed diseases   87-8, 89
   pronator teres syndrome   68
   radial tunnel syndrome   68
   tenosynovitis   62
writers' cramp   86, 87, 88
WYETH -V- THAMES CASE   129